DISEASE AND THREATENED BIRDS

Edited by
J. E. COOPER

Based on the Proceedings of a Symposium held at the XIX World Conference of the International Council for Bird Preservation, June 1986, Queens University, Kingston, Ontario, Canada.

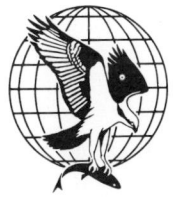

ICBP Technical Publication No. 10

Cover illustration: The Cockatiel (*Nymphicus hollandicus*) of the Australian interior. The species is one of many psittacines that may be susceptible to epizootic disease – a subject discussed by Steven McOrist in this volume.
Drawn by Trevor Boyer/Bernard Thornton Artists.

Copyright © 1989 International Council for Bird Preservation, 32 Cambridge Road, Girton, Cambridge CB3 0PJ, England.
All rights reserved.

British Library Cataloguing in Publication Data

Disease and threatened birds.
   1. Birds. Diseases
   I. Cooper, J. E. (John Eric) 1944–   II. International Council for Bird Preservation   III. Series   598.2'2.

ISBN 0-946888-18-3
ISSN 0277-1330

Prepared for publication by Anagram Editorial Service, Guildford, Surrey, England.
Typeset, printed and bound in Great Britain by Page Bros (Norwich) Ltd, Norfolk, England.

INTERNATIONAL COUNCIL FOR BIRD PRESERVATION

ICBP is the longest-established worldwide conservation organization. Its primary aim is the protection of wild birds and their habitats as a contribution to the preservation of biological diversity. Founded in 1922, it is a federation of 330 member organizations in 100 countries. These organizations represent a total of over ten million members all over the world.

Central to the successful execution of ICBP's mission is its global network of scientists and conservationists specializing in bird protection. This network enables it to gather and disseminate information, identify and enact priority projects, and promote and implement conservation measures. Today, ICBP's Conservation Programme includes some 120 projects throughout the world.

ICBP provides expert advice to governments on bird conservation matters, management of nature reserves, and such issues as the control of trade in endangered species. Through interventions to governments on behalf of conservation issues, ICBP can mobilize and bring to bear the force of international scientific and popular opinion at the highest levels. Conferences and symposia by its specialist groups help to attract worldwide attention to the plight of endangered birds.

ICBP maintains a comprehensive databank concerning the status of all the world's threatened birds and their habitats, from which the bird *Red Data Books* are prepared. A series of Technical Publications provides up-to-date and in-depth treatment of major bird conservation issues, while monographs provide comprehensive information on specific or regional issues relating to bird conservation.

ICBP now has a membership scheme, the World Bird Club, and issues a topical quarterly newsletter, *World Birdwatch*.

ICBP, 32 Cambridge Road, Girton, Cambridge CB3 0PJ, U.K.
U.K. Charity No. 286211

CONTRIBUTORS' NAMES AND ADDRESSES

The names and addresses given below are those provided by the contributors, and should be used by readers wishing to contact them. In some cases these addresses differ from those given in the text.

GWYN ASHTON, MVSc., MRCVS, Veterinary Investigation Centre, Polwhele, Truro, Cornwall TR4 9AD, England.

PHOEBE BARNARD, BSc., Department of Zoology, University of the Witwatersrand, Johannesburg, PO Wits 2050, South Africa.

W. R. P. BOURNE, MA., MB., BCh., Department of Zoology, Aberdeen University, Tillydrone Avenue, Aberdeen AB9 2TN, Scotland.

JAMES W. CARPENTER, MS., DVM., U.S. Department of the Interior, Fish and Wildlife Service, Endangered Species Research Branch, Patuxent Wildlife Research Center, Laurel, Maryland 20708, USA.

GARY G. CLARK, PhD., Center for Disease Control, San Juan Laboratories, GPO Box 4532, San Juan, Puerto Rico 00936.

MARGARET E. COOPER, LLB., FLS., Solicitor, c/o 35–43 Lincoln's Inn Fields, London WC2A 3PN, England.

J. E. COOPER, BVSc., DTVM., CertLAS., MRCPath., FIBiol., FRCVS., Royal College of Surgeons of England, 35–43 Lincoln's Inn Fields, London WC2A 3PN, England.

W. R. HANSEN, PhD., National Wildlife Health Research Center, U.S. Fish and Wildlife Service, Madison, Wisconsin 53711, USA.

NIGELLA HILLGARTH, BA., Department of Zoology, South Parks Road, Oxford OX1 3PS, England.

D. BRUCE HUNTER, DVM., MSc., Ontario Veterinary College, University of Guelph, Guelph, Ontario N1G 2W1, Canada.

C. DAVID JENKINS Jr, BSc., Endangered and Non-game Species Program, N.J. Division of Fish, Game and Wildlife, P.O. Box 236, Tuckahoe, New Jersey 08250, USA.

C. G. JONES, MSc., c/o Forestry Quarters, Black River Aviaries, Black River, Mauritius.

STEVEN MCORIST, BVSc., MVSc., PhD., MACVSc., Veterinary Research Institute, Park Drive, Parkville, Victoria 3052, Australia.

YOUSOOF MUNGROO, BSc., Forestry Quarters, Black River Aviaries, Black River, Mauritius.

C. C. NORTON, Ministry of Agriculture, Fisheries and Food, Central Veterinary Laboratory, New Haw, Weybridge, Surrey KT15 3NB, England.

M. A. PEIRCE, PhD., FIBiol., 16 Westmorland Close, Woosehill, Wokingham, Berkshire RG11 9AZ, England.

Contributors

R. L. REECE, BVSc., MSc., FACVSc., MRCVS., AFRC Institute for Animal Health, Houghton Laboratory, Houghton, Huntingdon, Cambridgeshire PE17 2DA, England.

F. T. SCULLION, MVB., MRCVS., School of Veterinary Science, Dept. of Pathology, University of Bristol, Langford House, Langford, Bristol BS18 7DY, England.

BELINDA STEWART COX, BA., c/o D3 Praphai House, Soi Pattana Sin, Nang Linchee Road, Bangkok 10120, Thailand.

STANLEY A. TEMPLE, PhD., MSc., Department of Wildlife Ecology, University of Wisconsin, Madison, Wisconsin 53706, USA.

DAVID M. TODD, BSc., Forestry Quarters, Black River Aviaries, Black River, Mauritius.

CHARLES VAN RIPER III, PhD., Department of Wildlife and Fisheries, Biology and Co-operative Park Study Unit, University of California, Davis, California 95616, USA.

DOUGLAS M. WATTS, PhD., Department of Virology, NAMRU – 3, FPO New York 09527, USA.

CONTENTS

ICBP	iii
Contributors' names and addresses	iv
FOREWORD by Christoph Imboden, Director, ICBP, Cambridge	viii
EDITOR'S PREFACE by J. E. Cooper, Convenor of the symposium	ix

THE PAPERS

1	Avian Pathogens: Their Biology and Methods of Spread *R. L. Reece*	1
2	Detection of Pathogens: Monitoring and Screening Programmes *D. Bruce Hunter*	25
3	Exclusion, Elimination and Control of Avian Pathogens *W. L. G. Ashton & J. E. Cooper*	31
4	Microbiological Investigation of Wild Birds *F. T. Scullion*	39
5	The Role of Pathogens in Threatened Populations: An Historical Review *J. E. Cooper*	51
6	Some Diseases of Free-living Australian Birds *Steven McOrist*	63
7	The Significance of Avian Haematozoa in Conservation Strategies *M. A. Peirce*	69
8	Disease-related Aspects of Conserving the Endangered Hawaiian Crow *C. David Jenkins, Stanley A. Temple, Charles van Riper & Wallace R. Hansen*	77

9	Mortality, Morbidity and Breeding Success of the Pink Pigeon (*Columba (Nesoenas) mayeri*) Carl G. Jones, David M. Todd & Yousoof Mungroo	89
10	The Impact of Eastern Equine Encephalitis Virus on Efforts to Recover the Endangered Whooping Crane James W. Carpenter, Gary G. Clark & Douglas M. Watts	115
11	The Role of Birds in the Long-distance Dispersal of Disease W. R. P. Bourne	121
12	Monitoring Parasites in Wild and Captive Green Peafowl in Thailand N. Hillgarth, C. C. Norton, M. A. Peirce & B. Stewart Cox	129
13	Faecal Bacteria in Unhatched Eggs of Box-nesting Kestrels (*Falco sparverius*) Phoebe Barnard	135
14	Legal Considerations in the Movement and Submission of Avian Specimens Margaret E. Cooper	141
15	Conclusions J. E. Cooper	151
16	Appendix 1: Register of Laboratories and Reference Centres N. Hillgarth & J. E. Cooper	155
17	Appendix 2: Protocols for Screening Birds and Guideline Procedures for Investigating Mortality in Endangered Birds J. E. Cooper	185
INDEX		191

FOREWORD

by Christoph Imboden, Director,
International Council for Bird Preservation

When will the world wake up to the reality that conservation is, first and foremost, a *science*? For five years now ICBP has been producing its series of Technical Publications, and with this volume we pass into double figures. Small as the landmark is, I am delighted that we have maintained an output of two volumes a year, and I am particularly proud that this tenth volume should assemble a broad set of pioneering contributions to science, and to conservation *as* science. It has always been my wish that our Technical Publications should enhance the image of conservation by aspiring to the most rigorous levels of scientific exposition, and in this collection of papers on the role and management of disease in relation to threatened birds, the merging identities of science and conservation could not be more striking.

The problem of disease in the conservation of wildlife is gradually becoming recognized as a serious matter. We are starting to gain some important insights into the regulation of animal populations by disease, and it is the responsibility of conservationists to be fully aware of the influence pathogens can exert on the objects of their concern, both in the wild and in captivity. This book, based on the Proceedings of a symposium held at the XIX ICBP World Conference in Kingston, Ontario, in June 1986, will I hope be prescribed reading for many scientists working for the conservation of bird species and populations round the world; and I hope, too, that it will become a landmark in the study of pathology in relation to conservation.

John E. Cooper is not only editor but also instigator of this book, and but for him it simply would not exist. I should like to pay the warmest tribute to this dedicated, indefatigable pioneer of avian disease research. John has worked with a selfless enthusiasm to help the cause of conservation for many, many years, putting his medical skills and expertise at the disposal of all who sought them. He has performed many kind services for ICBP, but perhaps none as great as is represented here in this book. On behalf of ICBP, I thank him and his wife Margaret, who helped organize the symposium in 1986, most heartily for all their work in bringing this volume to publication.

EDITOR'S PREFACE

by J. E. Cooper
Royal College of Surgeons of England,
35–43 Lincoln's Inn Fields, London WC2A 3PN, England

The XIX World Conference of the International Council for Bird Preservation (ICBP) was held in Kingston, Ontario, Canada, in June 1986. For the first time at an ICBP conference a symposium was organized on the possible effects of disease on rare species. Entitled 'Disease and Management of Threatened Bird Populations', the symposium attracted an enthusiastic audience who heard presentations from nine speakers.

These Proceedings include the papers presented at Kingston, together with others relevant to the subject which have either been offered or solicited. In addition they incorporate two appendices: one a list of laboratories and reference centres, the other an outline of health screening techniques.

One problem that arose both at the symposium and in the editing of the Proceedings was the definition of 'disease'. Dr James Murray's *A New English Dictionary of Historical Principles*, published at Oxford in 1897, gave four definitions of the noun 'disease' and the first of these was, 'Absence of ease; uneasiness, discomfort, inconvenience, annoyance; disquiet; disturbance; trouble'. The second was rather more in keeping with current usage, and referred to 'A condition of the body, or of some part or organ of the body, in which its functions are disturbed or deranged; a morbid physical condition; a departure from the state of health, especially when caused by structural change'. The sixth edition of *The Concise Oxford Dictionary*, published 80 years later, defines disease as an 'unhealthy condition of body . . . or some part thereof'. It is clear therefore that the term can include physical injuries (trauma, electrocution, burns etc.), poisoning, nutritional deficiencies and developmental abnormalities as well as infections and parasitism. Many of the non-infectious factors are well-recognized causes of ill-health and death in wild birds—pesticides (poisons) for example—but insofar as these Proceedings are concerned, the term 'disease' is restricted to infectious and parasitic conditions. The range of organisms that may be involved is enormous: it includes viruses, chlamydiae, rickettsiae, mycoplasmas, bacteria, fungi, protozoa, and both internal and external parasites. In this text the terms 'micro-organism' and 'parasite' are sometimes used interchangeably. Other important definitions, such as 'infection', 'commensal' and 'pathogen' are explained in the opening paper by R. L. Reece.

The term 'threatened' was used, as defined by IUCN (International Council for Conservation of Nature and Natural Resources), to include species that are considered to be endangered, vulnerable, indeterminate, rare or insufficiently known.

The questions we asked and then endeavoured to answer at the symposium were as follows:
1) What evidence is available on the role of disease or infection in threatened bird populations?
2) If a danger exists, is it likely to arise as a result of exotic pathogens?
3) To what extent can populations be monitored for evidence of disease or pathogens?
4) How can the risk of disease introduction and/or spread be minimized?

The answers to these questions are not all to be found in this volume—much still remains to be learned of the interaction between wild birds and the various micro-organisms and parasites that live on or within them—but here for the first time data are brought together which will, we believe, help ornithologists and others to understand better both the actual and potential impact of pathogens and diseases on threatened bird populations.

Many people contributed substantially to the success of the symposium and to the production of these Proceedings. Our thanks are due to the staff of ICBP and to those colleagues and friends in Canada who both provided hospitality and helped in the organization of the symposium. I am personally grateful to the Royal College of Surgeons of England for support and encouragement and to the staff of the Library of the Royal College of Veterinary Surgeons for their help with references.

The following have read manuscripts and provided valuable assistance with editing: J. R. Baker, N. C. Fox, A. G. Greenwood, I. F. Keymer, J. K. Kirkwood, J. C. Lewis, J. R. Needham, L. N. Payne, R. L. Reece, C. Riddell, V. R. Simpson and G. Wobeser. Sally Dowsett has given sterling service, by typing manuscripts and dealing with correspondence.

Finally I am grateful to my wife, Margaret Cooper, and my family for their support both in the organization of the symposium and in the editing of these Proceedings.

London
September 1988

J. E. COOPER

"More individuals are born than can possibly survive. A grain in the balance will determine which individual species shall live and which shall die . . . . The slightest advantage over those with which it comes into competition, or better adaptation in however slight a degree to the surrounding physical conditions, will turn the balance."

Charles Darwin
"The Origin of Species"
1859

AVIAN PATHOGENS: THEIR BIOLOGY AND METHODS OF SPREAD

R. L. REECE

AFRC Institute for Animal Health, Houghton Laboratory, Houghton, Huntingdon, Cambridgeshire PE17 2DA, England

ABSTRACT

There are many diseases of an infectious nature that can affect wild birds. This article contains definitions of many terms used in epizootiological investigations and contains some guidelines for the interpretation of field observations and case reports. Some of the salient features of avipoxviruses, avian influenza viruses, *Clostridium botulinum*, *Chlamydia psittaci*, *Pasteurella multocida*, *Salmonella* spp., *Aspergillus fumigatus*, coccidia, *Trichomonas gallinae*, ascarids and cestodes, and the diseases associated with them, are explained in such a way as to highlight differences in their biological characteristics and methods of spread. An understanding of these differences is important for the effective design and implementation of disease treatment, control and prevention programmes. Much of the information presented is derived from poultry diseases as the epizootiology of these has been determined. The principles are similar and application of them should reduce gaps in our knowledge of the epizootiology of many wildlife diseases.

INTRODUCTION

Friend (1981) proposed that there were four basic types of management response to wildlife disease problems; namely, fatalistic, frustration, fire-fighting and problem-solving. The biology and method of spread of different types of pathogens must be understood in order to allow the implementation of effective control programmes. It is vital to have such knowledge if we are to interpret correctly observations on diseases in avian species. This article provides some guidelines for possible methods of investigating such diseases, and gives examples of avian pathogens that have quite different biological characteristics and methods of spread. In this article the emphasis is on diseases of poultry because the epizootiology of these is more fully documented and better understood than is the case for many diseases of wild birds. Nevertheless, the principles involved are similar.

DEFINITIONS

A *pathogen* is an organism capable of causing disease.

Pathogenesis is the name given to the mechanism whereby a pathogen causes disease.

Infection is that state in which the body of one living organism, the host (in this context a bird) is invaded by another living organism. If this relationship is to their mutual benefit it is called *symbiosis*. If the host does not appear to be adversely affected it is a *commensal* relationship; the infection is said to be either *inapparent* (asymptomatic) or *subclinical*. The latter term is used to indicate that there may be subtle effects on productivity. The infected host is a *carrier*. If the host is harmed, the relationship is *parasitic* and the host has an *infectious disease* caused by a pathogen.

A *contagious* infection is one in which the agent is transmitted by close contact between an infected bird and a susceptible host.

A bird that is free of all associated organisms is *germfree*. If the associated organisms are known, it is a *gnotobiotic* bird. *Specific pathogen-free* birds are, as the name suggests, free from specified pathogens; other organisms associated with them are not defined. These terms are usually restricted to animals kept in laboratories.

Saprophytic organisms obtain their nutrients from decaying plant and animal matter.

Symptoms are subjective changes in the body or bodily function which indicate disease. The more appropriate term to describe the course of a disease as observed in affected birds, is *clinical signs*. Unfortunately, the clinical signs exhibited by affected birds do not always directly indicate the aetiology (Levine 1987). The typical 'sick' bird is depressed, inappetent, has a hunched-up appearance and ruffled feathers.

Disease is not synonymous with infection. In many cases, birds are infected with potential pathogens yet they are not diseased. Some reasons for this are because the *impact* of an infection is due to an *interaction* between the pathogen and the host in a particular environment. Similar pathogens may have different virulence and/or trophism characteristics. The spread from bird to bird may involve different methods and vectors, thus altering the infectious dose rate and route of infection. Birds of a certain age, or of particular strains or breeds, may be more resistant, or susceptible, to a particular disease. General immune-competence, specific immunity, intercurrent diseases and physiological state (e.g. egg-laying) may alter the birds' response to infection. Population density, nutrition, shelter, humidity, temperature and other environmental factors may modify that response and thus alter the outcome of infection. Examples of these phenomena are in the following text.

Treatment of any infectious or parasitic disease with appropriate chemotherapeutic agents and general nursing may suppress clinical disease and/or markedly reduce the population of susceptible pathogens in the host. Treatment does not usually eliminate carriers.

There are several ways in which the word *disease* may be used (Editor's Preface). First, disease may be a characteristic set of clinical signs and pathological findings, such as yolk sac infection, paratyphoid, Newcastle disease. Secondly, disease may be impaired physiological and/or bodily function, such as broken leg, oviduct impaction, slipped gastrocnemius tendon. Thirdly, a flock of birds can be said to be diseased if they have less-than-optimal performance

(Osborne 1963), or are considered to have abnormal characteristics for that particular species or strain. In this case disease is determined by a comparison with qualitative and/or quantitative data which are considered normal or desirable, such as growth rate, weight for age, rate of egg laying, feathering patterns, feeding behaviour. In wild birds this latter definition can encompass many important survival traits.

A disease may be defined in terms of its aetiology, its pathogenesis and/or its manifestations.

Diagnosis, from 'diagignoskein' (Greek—to discern), is the art or act of determining the nature of a disease. It is an interpretation of history, clinical signs, pathological findings, and the results of relevant laboratory tests. A tentative diagnosis may be modified in the light of further results, occurrence of further cases in the flock/group and/or the response (or lack of it) to specific treatments. The value of a correct diagnosis is that it provides impetus for those concerned with management (e.g. Government agencies and conservation bodies) to take appropriate action for the treatment, control and/or prevention of the disease concerned. Therefore the diagnosis must be accurate and meaningful. It may also need to be made swiftly, which has implications for the competence and experience of those investigating the disease, whether veterinarians or not. Publications such as those by Friend (1987), Wobeser (1981) and Cooper (1978) are important in this regard.

R. Koch (1843–1910) was a German bacteriologist who proposed that for a disease to be causally linked to an infectious agent, four conditions had to be fulfilled. These are known as *Koch's postulates* and may be summarized thus:

1. The agent has to be present in all cases of the disease, and to be absent from non-cases.
2. The agent has to be isolated and cultured in pure form.
3. Animals experimentally infected with the pure cultured agent have to develop the disease, identical in all respects to the natural cases.
4. The agent has to be reisolated from the experimentally infected animals.

Some apparently infectious diseases are unable to fulfill these conditions. Psittacine beak and feather dystrophy/French moult (McOrist, this volume) is a case in point where the disease has long been suspected of being infectious. Recently the disease has been experimentally reproduced. Although a virus-like particle has been regularly observed in association with natural and experimental cases, it has not yet proved possible to isolate and culture the causative agent (Wylie & Pass 1987).

The postulates proposed by Evans (1979) are less restrictive, and take into account causal associations between pathogens and hosts under specified environmental conditions, and allow for statistical comparison between infected (test) and non-infected (control) groups. They also accept a spectrum of host responses from mild to severe disease, following infection.

THE ROLE OF DISEASE

The questions that need to be answered concerning any disease situation are: (a) What is known about this disease? (b) How serious is it? (c) How widespread is it? (d) Where did it come from? (e) Will it persist? and (f) What are the implications?

Friend (1976) noted that there was a general lack of conclusive documentation

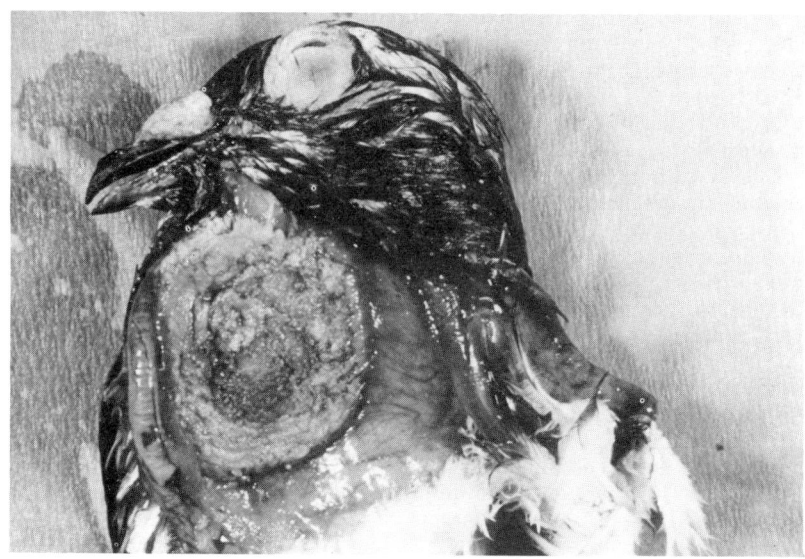

Figure 1: A large ulceration in the upper oesophagus of a Domestic Pigeon (*Columba livia*), caused by the protozoon *Trichomonas gallinae* (canker). (*Photo:* Reece)

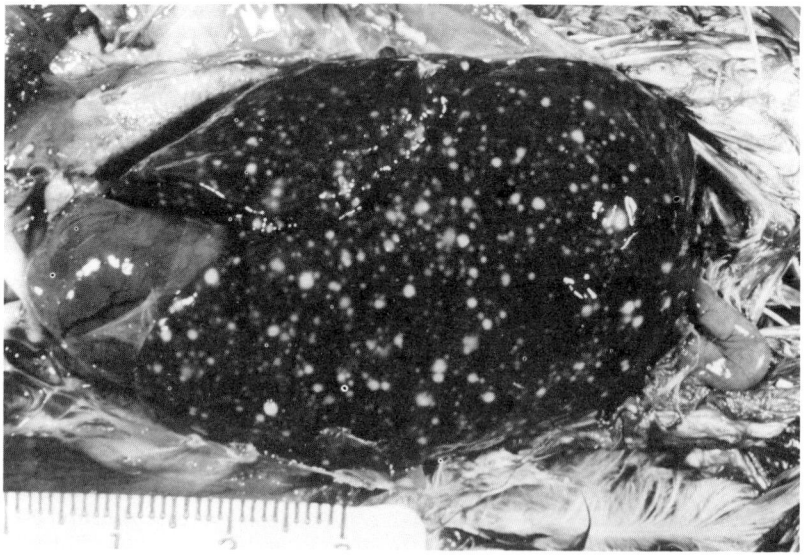

Figure 2: Greatly enlarged liver of a Common Bronze-wing (Pigeon) (*Phaps elegans*), showing numerous small (yellow) abscesses caused by the bacterium *Yersinia pseudotuberculosis*. (*Photo:* Reece)

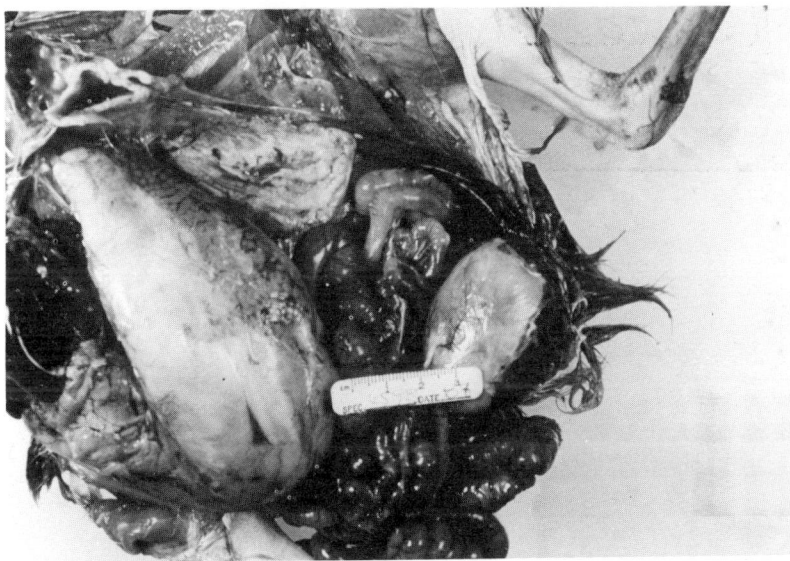

Figure 3: Thickening of the abdominal airsac of an Ostrich (*Struthio camelus*) due to diffuse fungal infection. (*Photo:* Reece)

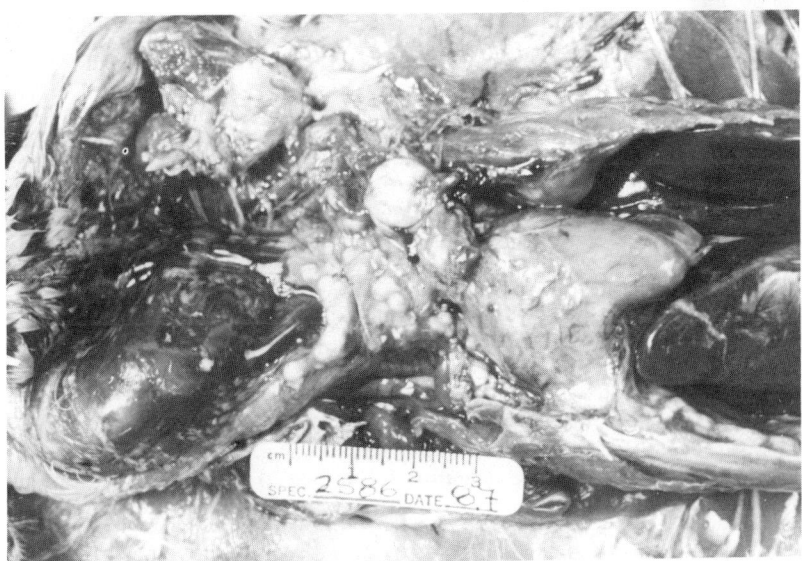

Figure 4: Nodular fungal infections in the thoracic airsac of a juvenile Little Penguin (*Eudyptula minor*). (*Photo:* Reece)

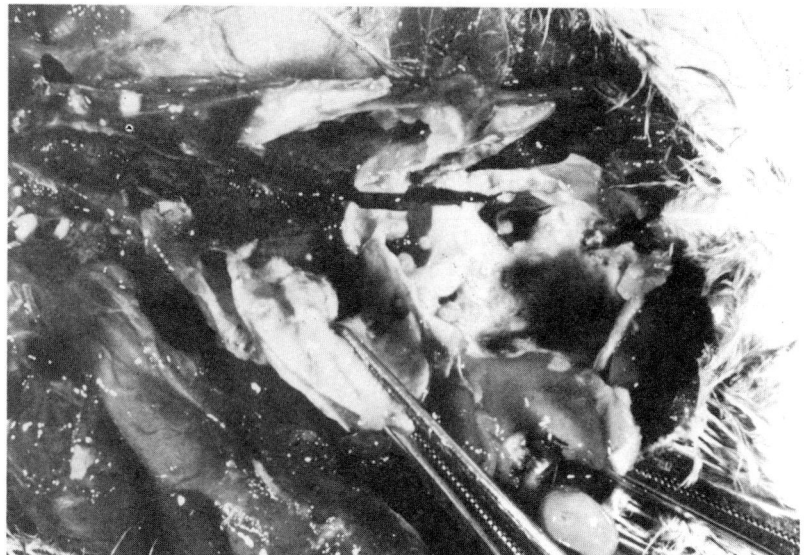

Figure 5: Velvety fungal fruiting bodies in the abdominal airsac of a Stone Curlew (*Burhinus oedicnemus*). (*Photo:* Reece)

of the role of disease in the population dynamics of wildlife. This still holds true. An increased understanding of a particular disease or the general disease status of any given population may derive from a series of successive approximations without a planned survey of definitive statistical design (Burton 1985). Such spot checks are often useful monitors of disease activity rather than providers of disease incidence data. Estimates of disease incidence in wild bird populations may be extrapolated from field observations of disease prevalence, detailed case studies, the results of experimental studies and/or the incidence of similar diseases in the same or other species. However, there is limited experience in effectively transforming such data into practical methods of disease control.

Reports of the incidence of diseases in avian species need to be interpreted with some caution. Necropsy findings on racing pigeons and doves differed in prevalence in the report by Reece (1987). The racing pigeons were specimens selected from over 100 lofts for the investigation of flock morbidity/mortality problems and poor racing performance, whereas the doves were natural deaths from two large 'healthy' bird collections over a ten-year period. Schlumberger (1956) studied 50 chromophobe pituitary tumours in the Budgerigar (*Melopsittacus undulatus*) and although there are grounds for suspicion that this species has a high incidence of this neoplasm, the specimens examined were specifically solicited from throughout the United States of America. The size of the population from which they were selected was not known.

Sometimes an *aetiological diagnosis* is ascribed to a disease in one species because it resembles a disease about which more is known in another species. However, in such cases a *morphological diagnosis* is preferable. The literature abounds with descriptions of Marek's disease and lymphoid leukosis in non-gallinaceous birds (for example Wadsworth *et al.* 1981). The association of such neoplasms with Marek's disease virus and avian leukosis virus is unknown and they would be better described as lymphoproliferative disease, lymphocytosis or lymphoblastic sarcoma. Neumann & Kummerfeld (1983) have recently shown that many adult budgerigars with kidney tumours and lymphoproliferative diseases, as well as apparently normal budgerigars, have group specific antigen to avian leukosis virus in their sera, but the significance of this observation is not known. 'Perosis' is another common diagnosis in birds, but slipped (luxated) gastrocnemius tendons is the better descriptive term. Perosis is a specific condition associated with dietary deficiencies—namely manganese, zinc, choline, biotin, nicotinic acid and folic acid—where there is a chondrodystrophy manifested by an increased width but decreased length of the proximal physes of the tarsometatarsus (Wise *et al.* 1973).

PRINCIPLES OF FLOCK INVESTIGATIONS

The number of diseased birds in a population is the *morbidity frequency*. This may be expressed as prevalence or incidence: the *prevalence* rate is a measure of the number of affected birds at a particular point of time; the *incidence* rate is a measure of the number of new cases occurring in a population over a stated period of time. These terms are often used incorrectly. In both cases the denominator is the number of birds, flocks or groups at risk (Thrushfield 1986). It is sometimes possible to extrapolate from prevalence data and obtain approximate information on the incidence of a disease. However, the incidence of various diseases in avian species, including the intensive poultry industry, is largely unknown. This makes it difficult to determine the impact of any particular disease.

In an investigation of a flock or group disease problem it is usually possible to develop a short-list of possible diagnoses based on history, observation and experience. A closer examination, collection of relevant samples and/or necropsy of birds with particular clinical signs may help to eliminate or retain some possibilities. Thereafter, it may be desirable to collect samples for testing, such as faecal swabs for bacterial culture, sera for serology, tracheal swabs for virus isolation and faeces for parasitology (Hunter, this volume). The number of samples to be collected and tested is dependent upon:

1. The test specificity and sensitivity.
2. The coincidence limit that is accepted for the test procedure, usually 95%.
3. The expected prevalence of infection in the flock being investigated.
4. The estimated population of the flock.

Tables indicating *sampling rates* can be devised or obtained from publications (Canon & Roe 1982; Eloit & Koutchoukal 1984; *Table 1*, this paper).

There are four types of results following any testing procedure (especially serological tests), namely: (a) test positive in an infected bird; (b) test negative in an infected bird; (c) test positive in a non-infected bird; and (d) test negative in a non-infected bird (Trajstman 1979; *Table 2*). These factors are often expressed as percentages but they are more correctly probabilities. Unfortunately the names given to them are not always consistent! The confidence with which a testing procedure is used, and the results acted upon, is greatly influenced by these factors. Many testing procedures are evaluated against each other rather than against the status of infection, and this can create difficulties in interpretation. No biological test procedure is 100 percent accurate (Baldock 1987).

Selection of specimens for detailed examination, particularly necropsy, can

Table 1: Number of birds to be randomly sampled to have a 95% chance of having at least one positive in the group sampled.

Flock size	No. of birds to be sampled						
	Disease prevalence						
	0.1%	1%	5%	10%	20%	50%	90%
100	–	95	45	26	14	5	2
500	–	225	60	30	14	5	2
1,000	950	260	60	30	14	5	2
5,000	2,250	300	60	30	14	5	2
10,000	2,600	300	60	30	14	5	2

Source: I. Morgan, personal communication.

Table 2: Possible relationship of the infection status and the results of testing procedures.

	Test result	
Host status	Positive	Negative
Infected	A	B
Non-infected	C	D

Notes: 1. Ability of test procedure to detect infected bird (sensitivity) $= \dfrac{A}{A + B}$

2. Ability of test procedure to detect non-infected bird (specificity) $= \dfrac{D}{C + D}$

3. Prevalence $= \dfrac{A + B}{A + B + C + D}$

4. Efficiency of test procedure = Specificity + (Specificity − Sensitivity) × Prevalence.

lead to apparent anomalies. Jordan (1956) noted a difference in the findings on birds from farms he was investigating, compared with findings on birds from similar flocks, submitted by their owners to a veterinary laboratory. Careful planning of surveys and studies is imperative if the data are to be of value. Case studies can be very misleading, but in wildlife disease investigations that is commonly the only type of data available.

In any disease investigation it is important to know the normal natural death rate, and its cause. For broiler chickens a useful 'rule of thumb' is that 0.5 to 1.0 percent of the chicks will die or be culled in the first week, with a third of that number being due to yolk sac infections and another third due to non-starter/starve-out syndrome. The peak prevalence of these losses will be between three and five days of age, therefore in a flock of 10,000 chicks, on day four there could be 10–15 chicks dead from yolk sac infections and a further 10–15 with starve-out syndrome, plus a few with systemic infections, congenital abnormalities and accidents. However, the flock as a whole can be considered 'healthy'. In a flock with a problem due to yolk sac infection the incidence of affected chicks up to two weeks old may be 10–20 percent; the clinical signs and pathology are the same in each case. In a 'healthy' broiler chicken flock the acceptable mortality rate is 0.5 percent per week in subsequent weeks with a slight increase after five to six weeks.

In commercial ducks and gamebirds, slightly higher mortality rates are often tolerated (2 percent in the first week, and thereafter 1 percent per week). For pullets reared on litter, 10 percent will have died or been culled by 18 weeks of age, and for caged laying hens the mortality and culling rate could be 0.5–1.0 percent per month. For free-living adult raptors, Newton (1979) reported that the annual death rate was 19–31 percent in Buzzards (*Buteo* spp.) and 49–57 percent in European Sparrowhawks (*Accipiter nisus*). The causes of death in a group of trained raptors have been documented (Kenward 1981). Such figures have to be borne in mind in any disease investigation. More data are needed for free-living birds.

Post-mortem examinations may reveal a great variety of diseases, but on many occasions there are no significant findings at all. Results of studies on broiler chickens (Hemsey 1965; Jackson *et al.* 1972; Blaxland & Borland 1977; Reece & Beddome 1983), broiler breeders (Jones *et al.* 1978; Reid *et al.* 1984a) and caged layers (Grimes 1975; Randall *et al.* 1977) have been published. There are many case reports of disease outbreaks among wild birds and ornithological collections (Cooper, this volume), but there are few published reports such as that by Kaneene *et al.* (1985) which gives details of causes of mortality and morbidity in apparently normal 'zoo' flocks. Many zoos and captive breeding programmes have such data which should be published so as to assist others concerned with these species.

A SAMPLE CASE

A case history of infectious laryngotracheitis (ILT) in laying hens in Victoria, investigated by the author, will be used as a basis to discuss some of the different ways prevalence and incidence data can be obtained, and to indicate problems that may arise. Farm A had 40,000 laying hens divided amongst six sheds. Within each shed the strains varied. Thus, in shed 1 there were 3000 WLAO strain X pullets reared on Farm A, 3500 WLAO strain Y pullets reared on Farm C, and 300 WLAO strain X pullets reared on Farm D. There were 20,000 laying hens in four sheds on Farm B and they were actually closer to shed 1 Farm A, than the other sheds on Farm A. The pullets were placed in shed 1, Farm A at 18 weeks of age.

The birds were clinically healthy until 24 weeks of age. At that time 10–15 pullets (strain X, ex Farm D) showed oculo-nasal discharge, swollen sinuses, poor appetite and respiratory distress. By 14 days, 200 pullets in this group had died, and of the remaining 100, 70 were moribund and the other 30 were apparently recovering. These pullets had not been vaccinated against ILT, and there were probably carriers of virulent ILT virus on the farm. The prevalence of ILT in this group was zero the day before the outbreak, 15/300 (0.05) on the first day and 70/100 (0.7) on the 14th day. The incidence was probably 100 percent during the two week period, but in a dynamic infectious disease situation at any one time it is possible to have susceptible birds that are unaffected, birds incubating disease, birds affected with disease showing mild to severe clinical signs, birds recovering from recent disease, birds that are carrying the pathogen yet are unaffected, and birds that are resistant to infection and free of the pathogen.

If, however, those pullets had been introduced into a free-range flock so that their identity as a group was lost, the following scenario may have occurred. Some time after 6800 pullets were introduced into the flock (total now 60,000 birds) the daily mortality rate increased from the expected 20/day (1 percent per month) to 40 per day. The animal attendants reported several small groups of sick hens, but most of the flock appeared healthy. Post-mortem examinations of dead birds revealed that about half of them had lesions consistent with ILT; moreover, these all appeared to be young pullets. Necropsy of birds with severe respiratory distress revealed similar lesions. The prevalence of moribund pullets would have varied from 0.002 (15/6800) to 0.01 (70/6600) or, if considered over the whole flock, at its peak there would have been 0.1 percent birds affected (70/60,000) (P = 0.001 during one month). The fact that all affected birds were one distinct group cannot be ascertained from this information.

Such scenarios could readily occur in wild bird populations with intermingling of groups with totally different histories; some being susceptible to certain pathogens and others being carriers. Investigation of such diseases often will be hampered by prevalence data, i.e. observations over limited time periods. Carcasses for necropsy examination may also have a high loss due to scavengers, predators and excessive autolysis.

Chlamydiosis, herpesvirus infection, mycoplasmosis, paratyphoid and avian cholera are more of a problem when birds are 'stressed'. As flocks or groups frequently harbour more than one pathogen, and a proportion of the flock or group may be more stressed than others due to laying/brooding, age, reduced feed intake or variable parasitic burdens, then there may be a greater incidence of a number of diseases in particular subpopulations.

METHODS OF SPREAD

Pathogens may be spread by vertical transmission, that is, contamination of the egg or embryo so that infection is passed to the next generation. This occurs with avian leukosis virus, reticuloendotheliosis, adenoviruses, *Mycoplasma* spp. and *Salmonella* spp.. Spread by horizontal transmission may involve inhalation of infective aerosols (e.g. Newcastle disease virus), ingestion of contaminated feed (e.g. coccidial oocysts), ingestion of an infected intermediate host (e.g. tapeworm cysticercoids in invertebrates), spread by vectors (e.g. spirochaetosis in ticks), direct contact (e.g. pox), and/or by environmental contamination of damaged tissues (e.g. erysipelas).

EXAMPLES OF PATHOGENS

Viruses

Viruses can multiply only in living (host) cells. There are many different types of virus that can cause infectious disease in avian species. They are classified on the basis of their nucleic acid content into DNA and RNA viruses, and within these groups the viruses may or may not have an envelope. The virus particles may be released by lysis (death and disruption) of the host cell, or by active budding-off from the cell membrane. The viral genome may be incorporated into host genes and thereby be transferred to progeny, as happens with avian leukosis virus. Alternatively the virus may infect a cell and not cause the death of that cell, thus creating a carrier. This is particularly common with herpesvirus infections. Enveloped viruses tend to be fragile and therefore require close contact between infected and susceptible hosts, and they often exhibit methods of spread dependent on carriers.

Poxviruses are naked (non-enveloped) DNA viruses. Avipoxviruses cause disease in domestic fowl, turkeys, quail, pigeons, canaries, sparrows, starlings, raptors, parrots and many other avian species (Matthews 1979). The various strains tend to be species specific in their host range; however, there are some antigenic similarities but not homology between turkey pox and fowl pox, and to a limited extent between canary pox and fowl pox (Tripathy *et al.* 1973). The genetic profiles of the various strains are very similar (Schnitzlein *et al.* 1988). There is sometimes cross-protection, for example pigeon pox is frequently employed as a mild vaccine to protect chickens from fowl pox (Tripathy & Cunningham 1984) and it has also been used in raptors (Cooper 1978). Parrot pox and fowl pox are also cross-protective, but quail pox is not (Winterfield & Reed 1985). Virulence of strains can also vary greatly. Pox viruses are very robust and will survive for long periods in the environment. The virus attacks epithelium, hence the commonest lesions are found on the skin. It is frequently spread by biting insects (mosquitoes and other Diptera) so the unfeathered areas of the head and legs are sites of predilection. Secondary lesions frequently occur due to spread of virus by preening. Humans can play a role in the spread of the virus. There is a report of venereal pox in turkeys which was spread by equipment used for artificial insemination (Metz *et al.* 1985). Infection can also occur following inhalation (diphtheritic pox).

Birds with cutaneous pox do not normally die, although affected birds may be inappetent and pyrexic. Diphtheritic pox is frequently fatal. In flocks of small passerines, pox of the tongue may be associated with significant mortalities. Immunity following infection is solid, and carriers are not normally considered to occur. However, immunity may not persist to the next season, particularly if infection occurs only intermittently. Avipoxviruses pose a serious threat to free-living birds (Jenkins *et al.*, this volume). Even if not fatal, pox infection can reduce viability and predispose affected birds to predation, secondary infection or accident.

The **avian influenza** (AI) viruses are enveloped RNA viruses classified according to their haemagglutinin (H1-13) and neuraminidase (N1-9). All AIs are type A group, and the accepted format of nomenclature is A/host/location/year(H,N) (Alexander 1982). Virulent AI in domestic poultry is sometimes referred to as fowl plague (Bourne, this volume), and it is a major concern to the poultry industry in many countries. The recent outbreak on one farm in Australia due to A/chicken/Victoria/85(H7N7) cost $A2.0 million to eradicate and there were incidental production lossess costing $A0.5 million/week (Carroll 1985). Large epizootics such as that in the United States of America in 1983–84 (A/chicken/Pennsylvania/83(H5N2)) cost many millions of dollars to control.

Avian influenza viruses are frequently isolated from free-flying birds, particularly waterfowl. There is a report of Common Terns (*Sterna hirundo*) dying of virulent AI (A/tern/South Africa/61(H5N3)) (Becker 1963) but in most other cases the viruses are isolated from apparently healthy birds. It should be noted that during the aforementioned outbreak of virulent AI in Australia, similar virus was isolated from Starlings (*Sturnus vulgaris*) on the infected farm and experimentally it caused 100 percent mortality in Starlings and 30 percent mortality in Sparrows (*Passer domesticus*) but no disease in Pekin Ducks (*Anas platyrhynchos*) (Nestorowicz *et al.* 1987).

The AI viruses replicate in the intestinal tract of carriers and are excreted in their faeces. The virus may then persist in contaminated water (dams, lakes) for several days. Often it is presumed that this is the method of spread of virulent virus to susceptible poultry. However, it is more probable that the AI viruses originating from wild birds are avirulent for poultry, and subsequently virulent strains are derived from these by selective adaptation, mutation, recombination or loss of defective interfering RNA viruses (Webster *et al.* 1984). Spread of virulent AI virus in affected poultry is probably by inhalation as it is associated with respiratory disease, whereas in wild birds avirulent AI virus is spread by the faeco-oral route (Alexander 1982).

The virulence of AI is due to a number of different genes. Antigenic *shift* is a major change in type occurring in a population, for example, in humans Asian flu (H2N2) was replaced by Hong Kong flu (H3N2) in 1968, which in turn was replaced by H1N1 in 1977. Antigenic *drift* is a detectable change within the H and/or N antigens (Laver 1982).

Bacteria

Bacteria are small unicellular organisms which normally can be cultured in or on appropriate artificial media. Most bacteria are saprophytes. Some are opportunistic pathogens which may cause disease under suitable conditions, such as wound infections and intestinal ulcerations. Only a few specialized bacterial pathogens, such as the *Mycoplasma* spp. and *Haemophilus* spp., are species specific in the host they infect. Other bacteria can infect and cause disease in a wide range of bird species and ages (Scullion, this volume).

Spores of *Clostridium* spp., including *Cl. botulinum*, will survive for many years in the environment, and under suitable conditions they will germinate. *Clostridium botulinum* is a saprophyte and will multiply in decaying vegetable and animal matter such as carcasses. Botulinum toxins A to G, of which C is most commonly associated with disease in waterfowl and other avian species, are produced in particular circumstances. The toxin is relatively stable and is absorbed following ingestion. The toxin can be isolated from the intestinal tract of maggots feeding on rotting carcasses. If this preformed toxin is ingested by a susceptible bird it causes flaccid paralysis typical of **botulism**. Thus botulism is not normally considered to be an infectious disease because it is caused by toxins produced by bacteria rather than by the bacteria themselves. However, there are some circumstances where *Cl. botulinum* can colonize the caeca and produce toxins which are then absorbed by the host (Miyazaki & Sakaguchi 1978).

Botulism or 'western duck sickness' kills millions of waterfowl in the USA each year, and there are occasional epizootics involving waders. Pheasants, quail and domestic fowl can be affected also. Smith (1976) noted that most major botulism type C epizootics were associated with prolonged warm weather, an increasing amount of stagnant shallow water, alkaline conditions, and accumulated rotting vegetation and dead aquatic vertebrates.

Although waterfowl and waders are frequently affected with botulism type C, there are few reports on their innate susceptibility relative to other avian species. Two hundred thousand LD_{50} mouse doses of botulinum type C toxin given orally were required to kill Chinese Spot-billed Ducks (*Anas poecilorhyncha*) (Ono *et al.* 1982). Four-week-old broiler chickens have an LD_{50} of 150,000 mouse doses of botulinum type C toxin given via the intramuscular route, and that is 2000 times the LD_{50} dose for twenty-week-old pheasants (Kurakzono *et al.* 1985). Turkey Vultures (*Cathartes aura*) were shown by Kolmbach (1939) to resist 100,000 times as much botulinum type C toxin as was required to kill a pigeon. It is not known if this difference was innate or acquired. However, it is not unusual to use virulent organisms to vaccinate young animals, including poultry, while they still have circulating maternal antibody, and that scenario could closely mimic the situation in carrion-eating birds and birds of prey.

Chlamydiae are bacteria which have a complex life-cycle requiring living host cells. The infective particle is not very robust, and under normal environmental conditions it will not persist for much more than a week or so. *Chlamydia psittaci* causes **psittacosis** in humans (and is thus a zoonotic disease) and in psittacine birds.

The disease is known as **ornithosis** in pigeons and ducks, and **chlamydiosis** in other species. It can cause abortion, disease of the reproductive tract, arthritis, encephalomyelitis, keratoconjunctivitis and/or pneumonia in various mammalian species. Subclinical enteric and respiratory infections are common. Field strains are known to vary in their virulence and other characteristics, and limited work has shown some differences in DNA between ovine, parrot and pigeon isolates (McClenaghan *et al.* 1984). However, isolates from one avian species will usually infect other avian species.

The method of infection is usually by inhalation of aerosols containing dried contaminated excreta. A carrier state with infection of the lower alimentary tract is common. Spread from one species to another is very probable.

The author has been involved in investigating outbreaks of chlamydiosis associated with deaths of juvenile and adult free-living Spotted Turtle Doves (*Streptopelia chinensis*), Peaceful Doves (*Geopelia placida*) and Domestic Pigeons (*Columba livia*), but chlamydiosis was not confirmed in flocks of supposedly affected wild psittacines.

Avian cholera (AC) is due to a systemic infection with particular strains of the bacterium *Pasteurella multocida*. It has long been recognized as a problem in domestic fowl, turkeys and gamebirds. Since the 1940s, AC has become a serious problem in migratory waterfowl (Windingstad *et al.* 1988) but probably all avian species can be affected with AC. In an affected flock, apparently normal birds may harbour virulent *P. multocida* in the choana (palatine cleft) (Curtis & Ollerhead 1981).

Infection is usually transmitted via the upper respiratory tract and conjunctivae. *Pasteurella multocida* will persist in the environment for up to two weeks after the removal of susceptible hosts. It frequently can be isolated from the upper respiratory tract of mammalian species such as cats, raccoons, pigs, cattle and humans. However, unless such strains have originated from disease in avian species, they are avirulent for birds under normal circumstances.

Immunity following infection will usually prevent clinical disease recurring due to that strain, but the birds remain carriers. They may be susceptible to disease due to other strains, and under conditions of stress such as overcrowding, reduced nutrient intake, other diseases, egg-laying, heavy environmental contamination, and introduction of the organisms into wounds (especially fight wounds), disease may occur.

The taxonomic position of *P. multocida* has been defined by DNA studies (Piechulla *et al.* 1985). There are several distinct systems which may be used to type *P. multocida* isolates but they are not comparable (Brogden & Packer 1979); moreover, although most virulent strains belong to capsular group A that is not the sole determinant of virulence.

Salmonella spp. are ubiquitous and under suitable conditions they can survive and multiply in the environment. They may be found colonizing the gastro-intestinal tract of most species of animals, including Antarctic birds (Oelke & Steiniger 1973). Under certain conditions, infection with *Salmonella* spp. may be associated with disease and this is called **paratyphoid**. This may vary from a mild enteritis to a systemic disease with polyserositis or petechial haemorrhages, or there may be localized infection such as meningitis, tenosynovitis, osteomyelitis or yolk sac infections.

Some of the *Salmonella* spp. which cause disease in humans also occur in birds. Unfortunately sewage and other effluents may contain human derived salmonellae which may then be transmitted to wild birds (Fenlon 1983). The number of salmonellae that establish themselves in the lower intestinal tract is affected by the

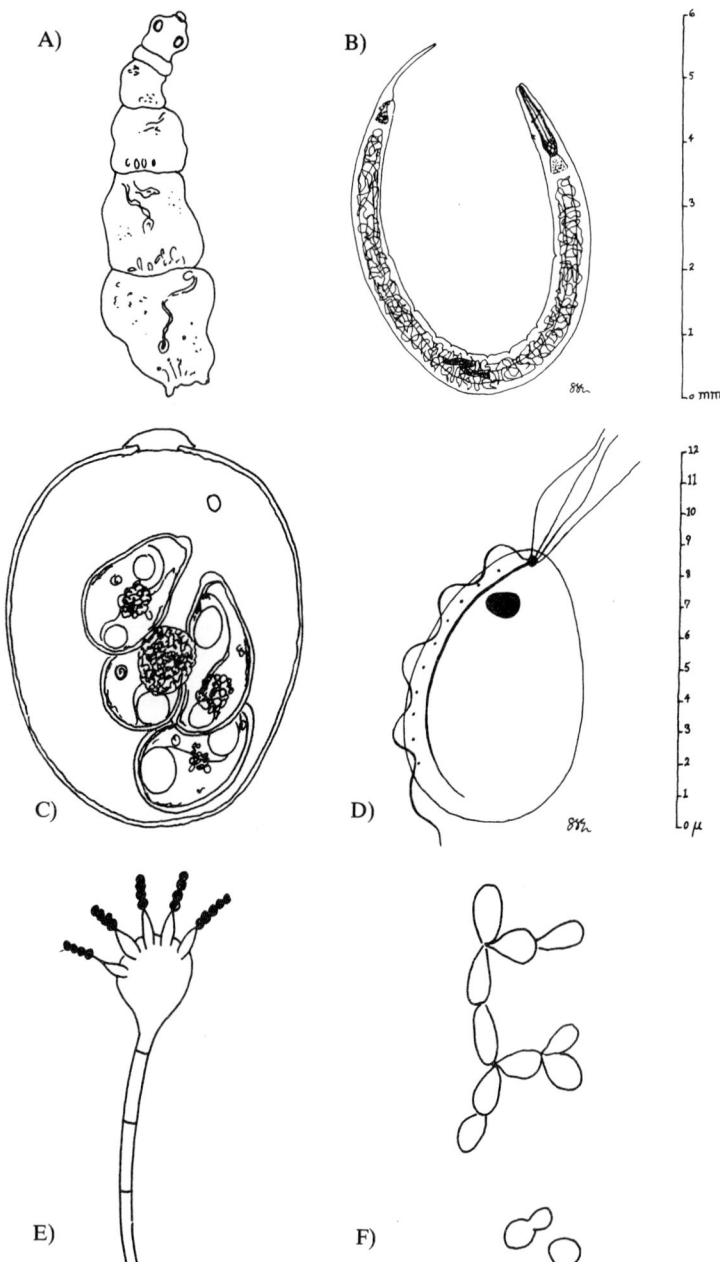

Figure 6: Composite illustration of some common avian pathogens. A) A cestode (tapeworm). B) A nematode (roundworm). C) A coccidial oocyst, greatly magnified. D) A flagellate protozoon. E) A fungus showing septate hypha and a fruiting body which is producing spores. F) A yeast (fungus). (*Drawings:* Samantha Elmhurst)

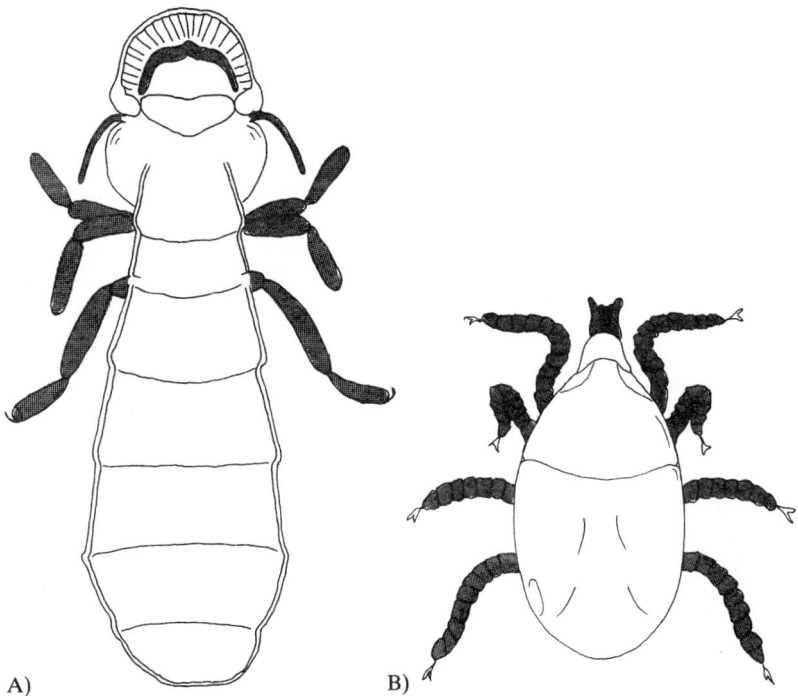

Figure 7: Two common avian parasites. A) A biting louse (Mallophaga). B) A parasitic mite. (*Drawings:* Samantha Elmhurst)

presence of other bacteria which influence pH, produce volatile fatty acids and occupy adherence sites (Schleifer 1985). This is the principle that underlies 'competitive exclusion', whereby known enteric flora are introduced into young domestic fowls so that their intestines are an unfavourable environment for the multiplication of salmonellae. Pathogenicity may be associated with penetration of the mucosal membrane lining the alimentary tract (Popiel & Turnbull 1985). In some cases infection may occur by inhalation. Localized infections are usually due to transport in macrophages (inflammatory cells) and deposition in areas of poor circulation.

Salmonella spp. can be classified by serotype, phage-type, antibiotic resistance patterns, plasmic profile analyses and biotype. These factors are not related to virulence (Poppe & Gyles 1987), but they are very important for epidemiological investigations. A recent outbreak of human paratyphoid was due to *S. typhimurium*, phage-type 12a. A similar strain had been isolated from chickens some months previously; however this latter strain had different plasmids and was therefore probably unrelated to the human disease episode (Anon 1987).

Apparently healthy adult birds may harbour salmonellae in the alimentary tract, and eggs that are laid will have varying degrees of salmonella contamination on their surface. These bacteria are motile and will penetrate the shell. Some developing embryos may die due to infection. If the chicks are subjected to environmental stress in the first few days of life, mortality due to systemic salmonellosis, i.e. paratyphoid, can be quite marked.

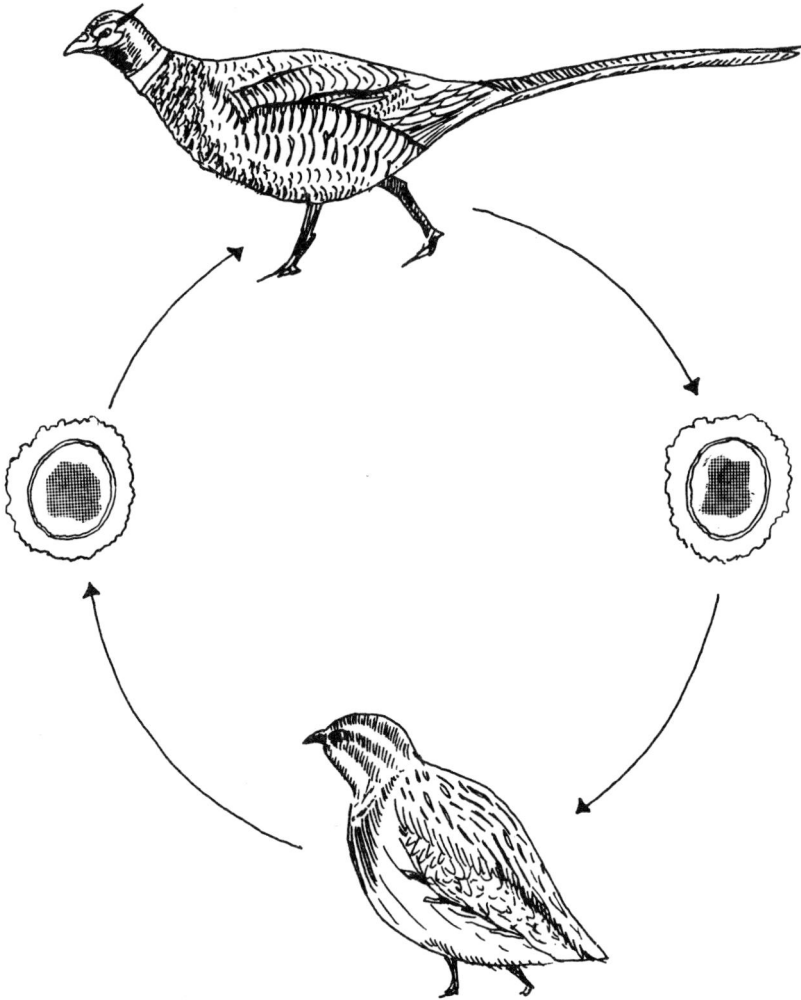

Figure 8: Life-cycle of a parasitic nematode of birds which does not require an intermediate host and can be transmitted from one bird to another. (*Drawing:* Samantha Elmhurst)

A flock or group of birds may become infected with salmonellae by vertical transmission, by contact with carriers (not necessarily of the same species), by ingestion of contaminated feedstuffs and/or drinking water. If the *Salmonella* spp. are pathogenic for that species and a sufficient number of organisms are introduced into the host, or multiply therein, and the appropriate predisposing factors are operative, then paratyphoid may occur. Paratyphoid is a common cause of death of recently imported and transported birds (Sawa *et al.* 1981). This has significant implications for disease control, especially in threatened species which may be captured and transported in order to establish captive breeding flocks.

Biology and Spread of Avian Pathogens 17

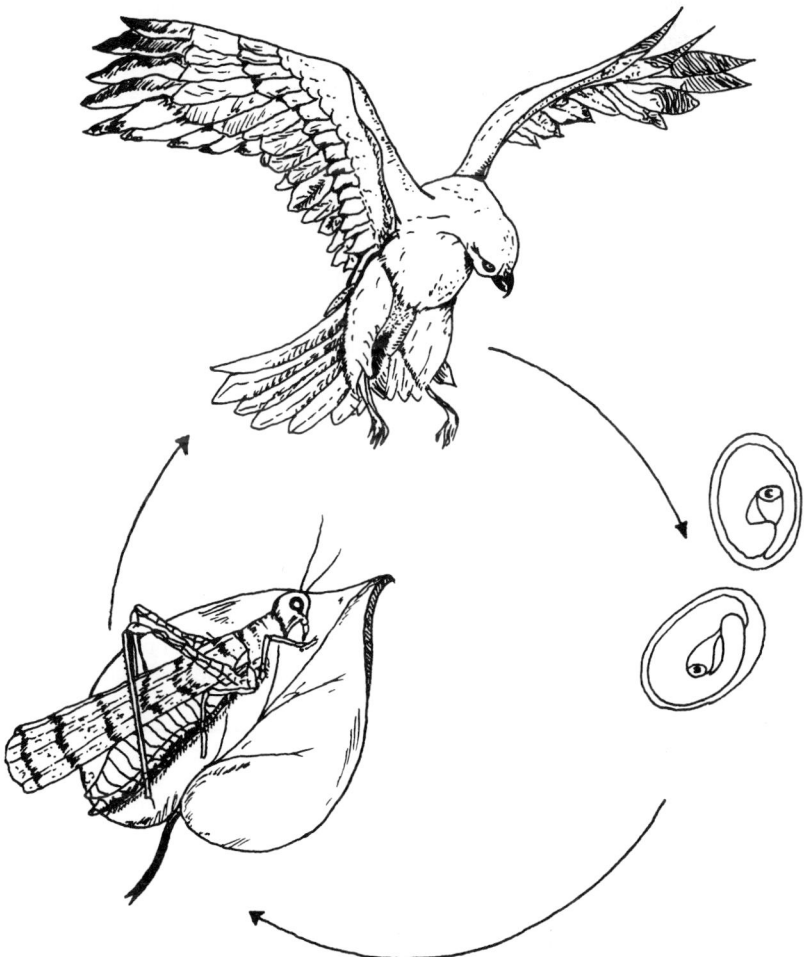

Figure 9: Life-cycle of a parasitic nematode of birds which requires an invertebrate intermediate host. (*Drawing:* Samantha Elmhurst)

Fungi

Fungi are simple plants which reproduce by means of budding and the formation of spores (except for the fungi imperfecti group which normally do not have a recognized sexual sporulation phase in the host). Most fungi are not pathogens.

Probably all avian species can be affected with fungal airsacculitis and pneumonia, usually due to infection with *Aspergillus fumigatus*. *Aspergillus* spp. are saprophytic fungi which are ubiquitous in nature. The disease is not contagious; that is, infection is not normally spread from bird to bird, but infection occurs because of inhalation of airborne spores (Chute & O'Meara 1958). Spores may be phagocytosed by alveolar macrophages and then be disseminated via the blood stream to the liver, brain, eye and elsewhere (Richard & Thurston 1983). The spores germinate and produce fungal hyphae which cause necrosis in the tissue and elicit a granulomatous inflammatory reaction. Fungal pneumonia is a common problem in captive birds and some wild birds, including raptors (Redig 1981), waterfowl (Stroud & Duncan 1982), penguins and psittacines (Reece, unpublished data). It appears to be more common in youngsters but this may be due to different exposure rates rather than age resistance.

Protozoa

Protozoa are unicellular organisms. Some can be cultured in artificial media; others require living host cells to complete their life-cycle. Saprophytic protozoa are ubiquitous.

Coccidia are protozoa which have a complex life-cycle involving asexual and sexual stages in living host cells. They normally affect epithelial cells of hollow organs such as the intestines, trachea, bile ducts or kidney tubules. The number of asexual and sexual cycles in the host is usually limited. The *Eimeria* spp. are host specific; thus *E. tenella* of domestic fowl is not a problem in other bird species. There are several reports of *E. tenella* in other species but these are considered doubtful by Reid *et al.* (1984b). On the other hand cryptosporidia (*Cryptosporidium* sp.) are probably capable of infecting fish, reptiles, birds and mammals, including humans (Tzipori *et al.* 1980). The oocysts of coccidia are very resistant. Specific environmental conditions are necessary before sporulation of the oocyst occurs: the sporozoites that are formed are the infectious stage and these have to be ingested by a susceptible host.

Trichomonas gallinae is a fragile flagellated protozoon with a simple life-cycle. It is the cause of a severe upper digestive tract disorder in pigeons and budgerigars ('canker'), and raptors ('frounce'). It has also been reported in other species. Strains of *T. gallinae* vary in their virulence. Trichomonads may be found in the pharynx of apparently healthy adult birds. However, when adult altricial birds feed their young, the trichomonads are transferred into the upper digestive tract of the hatchlings where they can cause severe disease. Clinical disease can also occur in adults and there may be transfer of trichomonads by direct oral contact, vomitus and contaminated drinking water. There are other morphologically similar, but unrelated, trichomonads in the lower digestive tract which can readily be confused with *T. gallinae*: investigation by an appropriate laboratory is necessary to be sure of a diagnosis.

Metazoan parasites

Metazoan parasites can be classified as external or ectoparasites (e.g. fleas, lice, ticks) and internal or endoparasites (e.g. respiratory mites, flukes, roundworms). Free-living birds can have heavy burdens of a variety of parasites. If superimposed on exhaustion and/or poor food intake, parasitism can be associated with death (Obendorf & McColl 1980). However, the contribution of the parasitism to the problem may be difficult to determine. Locke *et al.* (1964) reported extensive deaths (a 'die-off') in Mergansers (*Mergus serrator*) due to acute massive tissue invasion and destruction by larval *Eustrongylides* spp. (a roundworm) probably obtained from ingested fish.

Ascarid roundworms are usually found in the lumen of the small intestines. They have a simple and direct life-cycle. The eggs are discharged in the faeces and develop into the infective form after about two weeks. The infective eggs will remain viable under suitable conditions for up to a year, and may be carried about by earthworms and grasshoppers. Following ingestion by a susceptible host the larvae are liberated from the egg and take about four weeks to become adults and produce eggs. Heavy burdens may be associated with significant weight loss or

Table 3: Summary of biology and method of spread of some avian pathogens.

Pathogen	Persistence	Method of spread	Virulence factors	Host factors
Avipoxvirus	Robust.	Mechanical vectors; contact.	Some variation.	Species specific; strong immunity.
Avian influenza	Fragile.	Disseminated by carriers.	Antigenic shift/drift mutation, recombination—considerable variation.	All avian species, marked variation in species susceptibility.
Chlamydia psittaci	Fragile.	Disseminated by carriers.	Considerable variation.	Avian & mammalian species; stress exacerbation.
Clostridium botulinum	Spores survive for years; multiply in the environment.	Ingestion of preformed toxin.	Toxin production varies according to circumstances.	All avian species; marked variation in species susceptibility.
Pasteurella multocida	Poor survival away from bird.	Disseminated by carriers.	Considerable variation.	Any avian species; stress exacerbation; reasonable immunity.
Salmonella spp.	Multiplies in the environment.	Disseminated by carriers; ingestion of contaminated foodstuffs, water.	Many serotypes, phage-types, plasmid types; virulence varies.	All species in animal kingdom; stress exacerbation.
Aspergillus fumigatus	Multiplies in the environment.	Inhalation of spores.	Dose related.	All avian species.
Eimeria spp.	Oocysts robust.	Ingestion of oocysts; disseminated by carriers.	Trophism & virulence are E. species dependent.	Species specific; strong immunity.
Trichomonas gallinae	Poor survival away from bird.	Direct contact with carriers.	Some variation.	Many species; strong immunity.
Ascaridia spp.	Eggs robust.	Disseminated by carriers; some mechanical vectors; ingestion of eggs.	Dose related.	Broad host range; some immunity.
Cestodes	Cysticercoids persist in intermediate hosts.	Disseminated by carriers; investion of invertebrate host with cysticercoid.	Dose related.	Species specific.

emaciation. Damage to the intestinal mucosa may predispose to bacterial enteritis, and there may be mechanical obstruction of the intestinal tract. Some immunity does develop and parasite burdens tend to be greatest in young birds.

Ascaridia galli may affect gallinaceous birds, waterfowl, pigeons, psittacines and other avian species. *Ascaridia hermaphrodita* affects psittacines and other common aviary species, whereas *A. columbae* is usually restricted to pigeons (Shanthikumar 1987). There are at least ten species of ascarids reported from parrots (Mines & Green 1983).

On occasions, ascarid larvae from one species may invade the tissue of an abnormal host. Parasitic encephalitis due to migration into the brain of larval stages of the raccoon ascarid (*Baylisascaris pyocyonis*) has been reported in several species of birds including ratites, quail and partridges (Evans & Tangredi 1985).

Adult ascarids are found occasionally in abnormal sites such as the abdominal cavity or oviduct, and larvae may be found in the liver or lungs. Such aberrant parasites may be detected during routine post-mortem examination and are normally of little significance (Hunter, this volume).

Tapeworms (cestodes) have an indirect life-cycle involving a relatively restricted range of intermediate (invertebrate) hosts. Their final (bird) hosts are quite specific. For example, *Davainea proglottina* attaches to the mucosa of the duodenum of domestic fowl and heavy burdens can cause significant enteritis. The gravid proglottids (mature tapeworm segments) are released into the lumen of the intestine and discharged with the faeces. The hexacanth embryos (onchospheres) develop and are eaten by suitable intermediate hosts, in this case slugs or snails. The onchospheres penetrate the digestive tract and develop into cysticercoids in the body cavity. When affected slugs or snails are eaten by a susceptible host the cysticercoid is released and develops into an adult in about three weeks.

Enteric cestodes can cause deaths in small passerines (R. L. Reece, unpublished data) or they may be one type of parasite in birds dying from multifactorial causes or other diseases, as *Tetrabothius* spp. were in free-living Little Penguins (*Eudyptula minor*) in the work reported by Obendorf & McColl (1980).

CONCLUSIONS

Many organisms can infect birds and cause disease. Some diseases are associated with the death of individual birds. In the case of endangered bird species where individual birds are crucial, such diseases may be significant. Of more general importance are those diseases where large numbers of birds in a flock or group are affected. The biological characteristics and methods of spread of the pathogens used as examples in this article were chosen as they were quite different and the relative control procedures will therefore differ greatly (*Table 3*). No general recommendations for the control or prevention of avian diseases can be made until the pathogens responsible have been identified.

REFERENCES

ALEXANDER, D. J. 1982. Avian influenza—recent developments. *Vet. Bull.* **52**: 341–59.

ANONYMOUS 1987. Monthly report—April 1987. Salmonella Reference Laboratory, South Australia.

BALDOCK, F. C. 1987. Operating characteristics of diagnostic tests, interpretation of results and criteria for selecting a test. *Aust. Vet. Practit.* **17**: 126–30.

BECKER, W. B. 1963. The morphology of tern virus. *Virol.* **20**: 318–27.
BLAXLAND, J. D. & BORLAND, E. D. 1977. A survey of normal broiler mortality in East Anglia. *Vet. Rec.* **101**: 224–7.
BROGDEN, K. A. & PACKER, R. A. 1979. Comparison of *Pasteurella multocida* serotyping systems. *Am. J. Vet. Res.* **40**: 1332–5.
BURTON, R. W. 1985. Problems in disease survey design. *In:* Della-Porte, A. J. (ed.) *Veterinary Viral Diseases: Their Significance in South East Asia and the Western Pacific.* Academic Press, Sydney.
CANON, R. M. & ROE, R. T. 1982. *Livestock Disease Surveys: a Field Manual for Veterinarians.* Bureau of Animal Health, Department of Primary Industry, Canberra.
CARROLL, C. L. 1985. The virulent avian influenza outbreak Victoria 1985—key issues. *Proceedings 6th Australasian Poultry & Stockfeed Convention*, Melbourne.
CHUTE, H. L. & O'MEARA, D. C. 1958. Experimental fungus infections in chickens. *Avian Dis.* **2**: 154–66.
COOPER, J. E. 1978. *Veterinary Aspects of Captive Birds of Prey.* Standfast Press, Gloucester.
CURTIS, P. E. & OLLERHEAD, G. E. 1981. Investigation to determine whether healthy chickens and turkeys are oral carriers of *Pasteurella multocida*. *Vet. Rec.* **108**: 206–7.
ELOIT, M. & KOUTCHOUKAL, M. A. 1984. Sondage dans une population animale: estimation du taux d'infection des cheptels. *Epidémiol. Sante. Anim.* **6**: 61–73.
EVANS, A. S. 1976. Causation and disease—the Henle–Koch postulates revisited. *Yale J. Biol. Med.* **49**: 175–95.
EVANS, R. H. & TANGREDI, B. 1985. Cerebrospinal nematodiasis in free-ranging birds. *J. Am. Vet. Med. Ass.* **187**: 1213–14.
FENLON, D. R. 1983. A comparison of salmonella serotypes found in the faeces of gulls feeding at a sewage works with serotypes present in the sewage. *J. Hyg. Camb.* **91**: 47–52.
FRIEND, M. 1976. Wildlife diseases: philosophical considerations. *In:* Page, L. A. (ed.) *Wildlife Diseases.* Plenum Press, New York.
FRIEND, M. 1981. Waterfowl management and waterfowl disease: independent or cause and effect relationship. *Transactions 46th North American Wildlife Natural Resources Conferences.* Wildlife Management Institute, Washington.
FRIEND, M. 1987 (ed.). *Field Guide to Wildlife Diseases, Vol 1, General Field Procedures and Diseases of Migratory Birds.* U.S. Dept. of the Interior, Fish & Wildlife Service, Resource Pub. No 167, Washington D.C.
GRIMES, T. M. 1975. Causes of disease in two commercial flocks of laying hens. *Aust. Vet. J.* **51**: 337–43.
HARIHARAN, H. & MITCHELL, W. R. 1977. Type C botulism: the agent, host spectrum and environment. *Vet. Bull.* **47**: 95–103.
HEMSLEY, L. A. 1965. The causes of mortality in fourteen flocks of broiler chickens. *Vet. Rec.* **77**: 467–72.
JACKSON, C. A. W., KINGSTON, D. J. & HEMSLEY, L. A. 1972. A total mortality survey of nine batches of broiler chickens. *Aust. Vet. J.* **48**: 481–7.
JONES, H. G. R., RANDALL, C. J. & MILLS, C. P. J. 1978. A survey of mortality in three adult broiler breeder flocks. *Avian Pathol.* **7**: 619–28.
JORDAN, F. T. W. 1956. A survey of poultry diseases in mid-Wales. *J. Comp. Path.* **66**: 197–216.
KALMBACH, E. R. 1939. American vultures and the toxin of *Clostridium botulinum*. *J. Am. Vet. Med. Ass.* **94**: 187–91.
KANEENE, J. B., TAYLOR, R. F., SIKARSKIE, J. G., MEYER, T. J. & RICHTER, N. A. 1985. Disease patterns in the Detroit zoo: a study of the avian population from 1973 through 1983. *J. Am. Vet. Med. Ass.* **187**: 1129–31.
KENWARD, R. 1981. The cause of death in trained raptors. *In:* Cooper, J. E. & Greenwood, A. G. (eds.) *Recent Advances in the Study of Raptor Diseases.* Chiron Publications, Keighley.
KURAKZONO, H., SHIMOSAWA, K. I., SAKAGUCHI, G., TAKAHASHI, M., SHIMIZU, T. & KONDO, H. 1985. Botulism among penned pheasants and protection by vaccination with C1 toxoid. *Res. Vet. Sci.* **38**: 104–8.

LAVER, W. G. 1982. Variation in human and animal influenza viruses—molecular mechanisms. *Advances in Veterinary Virology*, Proceedings No. 60, Postgraduate Committee in Veterinary Science, University of Sydney.

LEVINE, B. S. 1987. Avian diagnostics: a guide to caring for caged birds. *Vet. Med.* (May); 469-81.

LOCKE, L. N., DEWITT, J. B., MENZIE, C. M. & KERWIN, J. A. 1964. A merganser die-off associated with larval *Eustrongylides*. *Avian Dis.* **8**: 420-7.

MATTHEWS, R. E. F. 1979. Classification and nomenclature of viruses. *Intervirology* **12**: 160-4.

MCCLENAGAN, M., HERRING, A. J. & AITKEN, I. D. 1984. Comparison of *Chlamydia psittaci* isolates by DNA restriction endonuclease analysis. *Infect. Immun.* **45**: 384-9.

METZ, A. L., HATCHER, L., NEWMAN, J. A. & HALVORSON, D. A. 1985. Venereal pox in breeder turkeys in Minnesota. *Avian Dis.* **29**: 850-3.

MINES, J. J. & GREEN, P. E. 1983. Experimental *Ascaridia columbae* infections in budgerigars. *Aust. Vet. J.* **60**: 279-80.

MIYAZAKI, S. & SAKAGUCHI, G. 1978. Experimental botulism in chickens: the cecum as the site of production and absorption of botulinum toxin. *Japan J. Med. Sci. Biol.* **31**: 1-15.

NESTOROWICZ, A., KAWAOKA, Y., BEAN, W. J. & WEBSTER, R. G. 1987. Molecular analysis of the hemagglutinin genes of Australian H7N7 influenza viruses: role of passerine birds in maintenance or transmission. *Virology* **160**: 411-18.

NEUMANN, U. & KUMMERFELD, N. 1983. Neoplasms in budgerigars (*Melopsittacus undulatus*) clinical, pathomorphological and serological findings with special consideration of kidney tumours. *Avian Pathol.* **12**: 353-62.

NEWTON, I. 1979. *Population Ecology of Raptors*. T. & A. D. Poyser, Berkhamsted.

OBENDORF, D. L. & MCCOLL, K. 1980. Mortality in Little Penguins (*Eudyptula minor*) along the coast of Victoria, Australia. *J. Wildl. Dis.* **16**: 251-9.

OELKE, H. & STEINIGER, F. 1973. Salmonella in Adelie Penguins (*Pygoscelis adeliae*) and South Polar Skuas (*Catharacta maccormicki*) on Ross Island, Antarctica. *Avian Dis.* **17**: 568-73.

ONO, T., AZUMA, R., KATO, T., TAKEUCHI, S. & SUTO, T. 1982. Outbreaks of type C botulism in waterfowl in Japan. *Nat. Instit. Anim. Hlth. Q.* **22**: 102-14.

OSBORNE, H. G. 1963. Teaching of clinical veterinary medicine. *J. Am. Vet. Med. Ass.* **142**: 888-94.

PIECHULLA, K., BISGAARD, M., GERLACH, H. & MANNHEIM, W. 1985. Taxonomy of some recently described avian *Pasteurella/Actinobacillus*-like organisms as indicated by deoxyribonucleic acid relatedness. *Avian Pathol.* **14**: 281-311.

POPIEL, I. & TURNBULL, P. C. B. 1985. Passage of *Salmonella enteritidis* and *Salmonella thompson* through chick ileocecal mucosa. *Infect. Immun.* **47**: 786-92.

POPPE, C. & GYLES, C. L. 1987. Relation of plasmids to virulence and other properties of salmonellae from avian sources. *Avian Dis.* **31**: 844-54.

RANDALL, C. J., BLANDFORD, T. B., BORLAND, E. D., BROOKSBANK, N. H., HALL, S. A., HERBERT, C. N. & RICHARDS, S. R. 1977. A survey of mortality in 51 caged laying flocks. *Avian Pathol.* **6**: 149-70.

REDIG, P. T. 1981. Aspergillosis in raptors. *In:* Cooper, J. E. & Greenwood, A. G. (eds.) *Recent Advances in the Study of Raptor Diseases*. Chiron Publications, Keighley.

REECE, R. L. 1987. Avian species. *Through the Naked Eye, Gross Pathology of Domestic Animals*. Proceedings No 97, Postgraduate Committee in Veterinary Science, University of Sydney.

REECE, R. L. & BEDDOME, V. D., 1983. Causes of culling and mortality in three flocks of broiler chickens in Victoria during 1979. *Vet Rec.* **112**: 450-2.

REID, G. G., GRIMES, T. M., EAVES, F. W. & BLACKALL, R. J. 1984a. A survey of disease in five commercial flocks of meat breeder chickens. *Aust. Vet. J.* **61**: 13-16.

REID, W. M., LONG, P. L. & MCDOUGALD, L. R. 1984b. Coccidiosis. *In:* Hofstad, M. S., Barnes, H. J., Calnek, B. W., Reid, W. M. & Yoder, H. W. Jr (eds.) *Diseases of Poultry*, 8th edition. Iowa State Univ. Press, Ames.

RICHARD, J. L. & THURSTON, J. R. 1983. Rapid hematogenous dissemination of *Aspergillus fumigatus* and *A. flavus* spores in turkey poults following aerosol exposure. *Avian Dis.* **27**: 1025–33.

SAWA, H., HIRAI, K., KINJO, T., SHIBATA, I. & SHIMAKURA, S. 1981. *Salmonella typhimurium* infection in imported passerine and psittacine birds. *Jpn. J. Vet. Sci.* **43**: 967–9.

SCHLEIFER, J. H. 1985. A review of the efficacy and mechanisms of competitive exclusion for the control of *Salmonella* in poultry. *World's Poult. Sci. J.* **41**: 72–83.

SCHLUMBERGER, H. G. 1956. Neoplasia in the parakeet: I spontaneous chromophobe pituitary tumors. *Cancer Res.* **14**: 237–45.

SCHNITZLEIN, W. M., GHILDYAL, N. & TRIPATHY, D. N. 1988. Genomic and antigenic characterization of avipoxviruses. *Virus Res.* **10**: 65–76.

SHANTHIKUMAR, S. R. 1987. Helminthology. *In:* Burr, E. W. (ed) *Companion Bird Medicine.* Iowa State Univ. Press, Ames.

SMITH, G. R. 1976. Botulism in waterfowl. *Wildfowl* **27**: 129–38.

STROUD, R. K. & DUNCAN, R. M. 1982. Occlusion of the syrinx as a manifestation of aspergillosis in Canada geese. *J. Am. Vet. Med. Ass.* **181**: 1389–90.

THRUSHFIELD, M. 1986. *Veterinary Epidemiology*, Butterworth & Co., London.

TRAJSTMAN, A. C. 1979. Diagnostic tests, sensitivity, specificity, efficiency and prevalence. *Aust. Vet. J.* **55**: 289.

TRIPATHY, D. N., HANSON, L. E. & KILLINGER, A. H. 1973. Studies on differentiation of avian pox viruses. *Avian Dis.* **17**: 325–33.

TRIPATHY, D. N. & CUNNINGHAM, C. H. 1984. Avian pox. *In:* Hofstad, M. S., Barnes, H. J., Calnek, B. W., Reid, W. M. and Yoder, H. W. Jr (eds.) *Diseases of Poultry*, 8th edition Iowa State University Press, Ames.

TZIPORI, S., ANGUS, K. W., CAMPBELL, I. & GRAY, E. W. 1980. *Cryptosporidium:* evidence for a single species genus. *Infect. Immun.* **30**: 884–6.

WADSWORTH, P. F., JONES, D. M. & PUGSLEY, S. L. 1981. Some cases of lymphoid leukosis in captive wild birds. *Avian Pathol.* **10**: 499–504.

WEBSTER, R. J., KAWAOKA, Y., BEAN, W. J. & NEAVE, C. W. 1984. Molecular characterization of the A/chickens/Pennsylvania/83(H5N2) influenza viruses. *Proceedings 88th Annual Meeting U.S. Animal Health Association*, Texas.

WINDINGSTAD, R. M., KERR, S. M., DUNCAN, R. M. & BRAND, C. J. 1988. Characterization of an avian cholera epizootic in wild birds in Western Nebraska. *Avian Dis.* **32**: 124–31.

WINTERFIELD, R. W. & REED, W. 1985. Avian pox: infection and immunity with quail, psittacine, fowl and pigeon poxvaccines. *Poult. Sci.* **64**: 65–70.

WISE, D. R., JENNINGS, A. R. & BOSTOCK, D. E. 1973. Perosis in turkeys. *Res. Vet. Sci.* **14**: 167–72.

WOBESER, G. A. 1981. *Diseases of Wild Waterfowl.* Plenum Press, New York.

WYLIE, S. L. & PASS, D. A. 1987. Experimental reproduction of psittacine beak and feather dystrophy/French moult. *Avian Pathol.* **16**: 261–81.

DETECTION OF PATHOGENS: MONITORING AND SCREENING PROGRAMMES

D. BRUCE HUNTER

Department of Pathology, Ontario Veterinary College, University of Guelph, Guelph, Ontario N1G 2W1, Canada

ABSTRACT

Much can be learned from the monitoring of wild birds, and appropriate precautions can be taken to exclude or contain potentially pathogenic organisms. Clinical and post-mortem techniques which can be used are discussed, amongst them haematological examination, serology and microbiological culture.

INTRODUCTION

The role of disease in free-living avian species is poorly understood. Although large-scale mortality of local populations is not infrequently reported, for example the 1973 'dieoff' of waterfowl on Lake Andes National Wildlife Refuge, South Dakota, due to duck virus enteritis (Friend & Pearson 1973) or the massive avian cholera outbreaks in California (Rosen 1971) and Texas (Jensen & Williams 1964), many biologists do not consider disease to be a significant factor in altering population dynamics (see Cooper, this volume). In commercial livestock production, however, the importance of infectious disease is well documented. Millions of dollars are spent annually on research into disease and the development of therapeutic and prophylactic health management strategies.

Disease may cause direct mortality but more commonly results in poor condition (unthriftiness) which may predispose birds to starvation or predation. Disease may also manifest itself in more subtle ways by altering reproductive success, reducing fertility or decreasing embryo survival, as documented for chemical pollutants such as polychlorinated biphenyls (Briggs & Harris 1973; Peakall & Peakall 1973; Gilman *et al.* 1977) and organochlorines—for example, DDT (Tucker & Haegele 1970; Kolaja 1977) and DDE (Longcore *et al.* 1971; Risebrough & Anderson 1975). The smaller the population base of the species and the more controlled its management, the greater is the potential significance of disease (Ashton & Cooper, this volume). Endangered or threatened species, and those managed in propagation and re-introduction programmes, are particularly at risk. The deaths in endangered Whooping Cranes (*Grus americana*) at the Patuxent Wildlife Research Center in Maryland, USA, caused by eastern equine encephalitis virus (Dein *et al.* 1986; Carpenter *et al.*, this volume), and mortality in a Burrowing Owl (*Athene cunicularia*) captive propagation project in Ontario, Canada, caused by the gapeworm *Cyathostoma americana* (Hunter et al. 1987), are examples of how disease can exert major effects on small, closely managed, populations of birds.

For many years the commercial poultry industry has established and used disease monitoring programmes in order (1) to ascertain the range of diseases or infectious agents present in their flocks, (2) to determine the significance of these agents in affecting flock production and survival, and (3) to set up prophylactic management strategies to solve or minimize the problem where it has a significant effect on recruitment, survival or production. Similar monitoring (screening) programmes can be used in wild birds. Field biologists, in cooperation with trained veterinarians, could and should make use of them—for example, during routine banding (ringing) sessions, at hunter check stations and in propagation projects. Monitoring programmes not only help to determine the prevalence of disease in free-living populations and in birds kept for captive breeding purposes, but also increase our knowledge of normal physiological parameters of various species.

MONITORING TECHNIQUES

Monitoring (screening) can be carried out on live or dead birds but the tests that are carried out may differ. The aim in both instances is to take representative samples which can be examined in the laboratory in order to provide information on the birds' health status.

An important prerequisite of monitoring live birds is thorough clinical examination (Appendix 2). This is followed or accompanied by the collection of samples. The investigation of dead birds involves necropsy (gross post-mortem examination) and supporting laboratory tests.

Haematology

Avian clinical haematology is a new and rapidly developing area of avian medicine. Small quantities of blood can be obtained easily and atraumatically from the caudal tibial vein, jugular vein or ulnar vein using a small gauge (25–27g) needle and capillary tubes. Although 8–10 percent of the blood volume of a bird can be taken without adverse effects, worthwhile information can be obtained from only two to three microcapillary tubes (200–300µl) of blood. Blood collected in the field for routine haematology can be collected in vials coated with an anticoagulant such as EDTA. If serum is required for biochemical or enzyme analysis or serology (see below), serum tubes containing no anticoagulant are used. The blood should be stored in an insulated cooler chest or on ice for analysis at a later time. Blood will clot in serum tubes within minutes, and the clot will retract after several hours allowing the serum to be removed by pipette. Incubating the clotted blood at 37°C for 30 minutes will often increase the serum yield. Serum should be frozen immediately and stored for later analysis. Blood smears should be prepared at the time of blood collection, air-dried and stored in slide boxes to prevent dust accumulation and scratching.

Changes in the type and number of cells in the peripheral blood will reflect changes in the body's physiological demands, the presence of inflammatory processes or disease states within the body, and the condition and hydration of the bird. Valuable tests include packed cell volume (haematocrit), total plasma protein and haemoglobin estimations, and white and red blood cell counts (Hawkey & Samour 1988). This information can provide valuable biological data about physiological changes which occur seasonally or during stress periods such as migration, moult and reproduction. Smears can be used to screen for the presence of haematozoa and other blood parasites (see later and Peirce, this volume) and to carry out differential white blood cell counts.

Serology

Serological examination can provide evidence of past or current exposure to specific disease-causing agents. A properly organized programme of serial blood sampling will help to determine both the presence and prevalence of exposure to a specific disease-causing agent within a population, patterns of horizontal (bird to bird) or vertical (through the egg) transmission of disease, including the potential of 'carrier' animals and the occurrence of active infection. The poultry industry routinely uses these techniques of 'flock profiling' or serial serology to monitor disease in both breeder and commercial flocks. In propagation and reintroduction programmes serological screening may be used to ensure that birds destined for release are unlikely to introduce disease into free-flying populations. It is also an important component of monitoring programmes for birds in quarantine—for example 'exotic' species being brought into a new environment.

Microbiological culture

Bacteria and viruses can be cultured on artificial media or within tissue culture or embryonated eggs. These procedures are routinely carried out in many private or governmental veterinary laboratories. Nasal swabs, pharyngeal swabs, faecal samples or cloacal swabs may be taken in the field and forwarded to diagnostic laboratories for culture. Special culture swabs are available that contain a nutrient medium that prevents the swabs from drying out prior to analysis. Studies on the epizootiology (epidemiology) of duck plague (duck virus enteritis), employing virus isolation techniques, have shown that the causative organism, a *Herpesvirus*, resides in a latent form within the nervous tissue of clinically normal carrier ducks and may be shed into the oral cavity and transmitted through the saliva and faeces during periods of stress (Burgess *et al.* 1979). This is similar to the pathogenesis of *Herpes simplex* infection (cold sores) in humans. Culture of cloacal swabs of migrating waterfowl has demonstrated the potential of these species in spreading avian influenza virus over long distances (Slemons & Easterday 1977). These and similar studies with other pathogens are essential if the natural history of disease in wildlife populations is to be studied fully.

Parasitology

External and internal parasites are common in most free-living avian species. The significance of many parasites is poorly understood but nestlings and fledglings are most likely to be most susceptible to pathogenic effects. During routine handling of wild birds—for instance, on nest counts and banding programmes—it may be possible to search for lice, mites or biting flies. These should be counted and identified. Blood smears can be made in the field, air dried, labelled and saved for examination in the laboratory for blood parasites. Parasites such as *Haemoproteus* spp., *Leucocytozoon* spp., and *Plasmodium* spp. are common in many species of birds (Levine 1971; Bennett 1982) but their disease-causing potential is poorly understood (Peirce, this volume). Faecal samples may be taken in the field (cloacal swabs) or collected from nests and saved in plastic freezer bags for examination in the laboratory. Techniques for performing wet mount examinations and faecal flotations are described in standard parasitology and veterinary diagnostic textbooks (Georgi & Georgi 1985).

Necropsy

A thorough post-mortem examination of all birds (free-living or captive) that die or are killed plays an important part in monitoring the occurrence of disease and the prevalence of pathogens. Gross post-mortem examination is followed by microscopical investigation of tissues and other supporting tests such as microbiological culture (Appendix 2). Standard necropsy techniques are well described (Wobeser 1981; Graham 1984; Lowenstine 1986) while useful guides for field ornithologists include those by Cooper (1983) and van Riper & van Riper (1980). A proper post-mortem examination should reveal any disease process including parasite infestation, and will permit the collection of samples of selected organs for analysis for environmental contaminants such as heavy metals and pesticides. The use of wildlife, particularly species at the top of the food chain, to monitor environmental chemical pollution is well documented.

CONCLUSIONS

Death prior to fledging and during the first year of life is prevalent in most avian species. There is a paucity of information on the factors that cause this mortality or that may predispose older birds to starvation or predation. Biologists, ecologists and wildlife veterinarians each have their specific areas of expertise, and these should be used co-operatively to help develop a truly 'holistic' approach to the study of population dynamics.

REFERENCES

BENNETT, G. F. 1982. *A Host-parasitic Catalogue of the Avian Haematozoa.* St. John's, Newfoundland, Memorial University, Newfoundland.

BRIGGS, D. M. & HARRIS, J. R. 1973. Polychlorinated biphenyls influence in hatchability. *Poult. Sci.* **52**1: 1291–4.

BURGESS, E. C., OSSA, J. & YUILL, T. M. 1979. Duck plague: a carrier state in waterfowl. *Avian Dis.* **23(4)**: 940–9.

COOPER, J. E. 1983. *Guideline Procedures for Investigating Mortality in Endangered Birds.* International Council for Bird Preservation, Cambridge.

DEIN, F. J., CARPENTER, J. W., CLARK, MONTALI, R. J., CRABBS, C. L., TSAI, T. F. & DOCHERTY, D. E. 1986. Mortality of captive whooping cranes caused by eastern equine encephalitis virus. *J. Am. vet. med. Ass.* **189**: 1006–10.

FRIEND, M. & PEARSON, G. L. 1973. *Duck Plague (Duck Virus Enteritis) in Wild Waterfowl.* US Bureau of Sport Fisheries and Wildlife, Washington DC.

GEORGI, J. R. & GEORGI, M. E. 1985. Antemortem diagnosis. *In:* Georgi, J. R. (ed.) *Parasitology for Veterinarians* Fourth edition. W. B. Saunders Co., Philadelphia, London, Toronto and Mexico City.

GILMAN, A. P., FOX, G. A., PEAKALL, D. B., TEEPLE, S. M., CARROL, T. R. & HAYMES, G. T. 1977. Reproductive parameters and egg contaminant levels of Great Lakes Herring Gulls. *J. Wildl. Manage.* **41**: 458–68.

GRAHAM, D. L. 1984. Necropsy procedures in birds. *Vet. Clin. North Am.* **14**: 173–7.

HAWKEY, C. M. & SAMOUR, H. J. 1988. The value of clinical hematology in exotic birds. *In:* Jacobson, E. R. & Kollias, G. V. (eds). *Exotic Animals.* Churchill Livingstone, New York and Edinburgh.

HUNTER, D. B., McKEEVER, K. & CRAWSHAW, G. 1987. Disease susceptibility in owls.

In: Nero, R. W., Clark, R. J., Knapton, R. J. & Hamre, R. H. (eds). *Proceedings of the Symposium on Biology and Conservation of Northern Forest Owls.* USDA Forest Service General Technical Report RM-142.

JENSEN, W. I. & WILLIAMS, C. 1964. Botulism and fowl cholera. *In:* Lindusky, J. P. (ed.) *Waterfowl Tomorrow.* US Government Printing Office, Washington DC.

KOLAJA, G. J. 1977. The effects of DDT, DDE and their sulfonated derivatives on eggshell formation in the mallard duck. *Bull. Environ. Contam. Toxicol.* **17**: 696–701.

LEVINE, N. D. 1971. A check-list of the species of the genus *Haemoproteus. J. Protozool.* **18**: 475–84.

LONGCORE, J. R., SAMSON, F. B. & WHITTENDALE, T. W. 1971. DDE thins eggshells and lowers reproductive success of captive black ducks. *Bull. Environ. Contam. Toxicol.* **6**: 485–90.

LOWENSTINE, L. J. 1986. Necropsy procedures. *In:* Harrison, G. J. & Harrison, L. R. (eds). *Clinical Avian Medicine and Surgery.* W. B. Saunders, Philadelphia.

PEAKALL, D. B. & PEAKALL, M. L. 1973. Effect of a polychlorinated biphenyl on the production of artificially and naturally incubated dove eggs. *J. Appl. Ecol.* **10**: 863–7.

RISEBROUGH, R. W. & ANDERSON, D. W. 1975. Some effects of DDE and PCB on mallards and their eggs. *J. Wildl. Manage.* **39**: 508–12.

ROSEN, M. N. 1971. Avian cholera. *In:* Davis, J. W., Anderson, R. C., Karstad, L. & Trainer, D. O. (eds). *Infectious and Parasitic Diseases of Wild Birds.* Iowa State University Press, Ames.

SLEMONS, R. D. & EASTERDAY, B. C. 1977. Type-A influenza viruses in the feces of migratory waterfowl. *J. Am. vet. med. Ass.* **171**: 947.

TUCKER, R. K. & HAEGELE, H. A. 1970. Eggshell thinning as influenced by method of DDT exposure. *Bull. Environ. Contam. Toxicol.* **5**: 191–4.

VAN RIPER, C. & VAN RIPER, S. G. 1980. A necropsy procedure for sampling disease in wild birds. *Condor* **82**: 85–98.

WOBESER, G. A. 1981. Necropsy and sample preservation techniques. *In:* Wobeser, G. A. (ed.) *Diseases of Wild Waterfowl.* Plenum Press, New York.

EXCLUSION, ELIMINATION AND CONTROL OF AVIAN PATHOGENS

W. L. G. Ashton[1] & J. E. Cooper[2]

1 Veterinary Investigation Centre, Polwhele, Truro, Cornwall TR4 9AD, England
2 Royal College of Surgeons of England, 35–43 Lincoln's Inn Fields, London WC2A 3PN, England

ABSTRACT

The movement of live birds, avian carcasses and eggs between countries and from one locality to another carries with it the risk of spread of a variety of avian pathogens. This trade cannot be stopped completely and will continue to present a health hazard to domestic and wild birds, humans and other mammals. A number of measures are needed to minimize the risk, and these must be thorough, sensible and continuous. Similar precautions can be used to help protect isolated populations of threatened birds.

INTRODUCTION

There are a number of important reasons why exclusion, elimination and control of avian pathogens are desirable. Many countries now have valuable and healthy national poultry flocks that are susceptible to a wide range of avian pathogens. Considerable effort and expense over a long period will have been incurred in improving the health of these flocks. In addition, avian pathogens such as *Chlamydia psittaci* and salmonellae are a potential threat to human health, and certain organisms can infect and cause disease in indigenous wildlife and in animals, including threatened birds, kept in zoos and captive breeding programmes.

The ways in which avian pathogens can be introduced into a country, or a population, will be considered. In the first section particular emphasis is laid upon poultry and, to a certain extent, captive non-domesticated birds since it is here that most work has been done. The possible applications to threatened birds are discussed in the second part.

IMPORTATION OF LIVE BIRDS

If a country is fortunate enough to have a poultry or wild bird population, captive or free-living, that is free of significant avian pathogens, every effort will be made to maintain its satisfactory health status. Infectious agents can be readily introduced into a country by the importation of live birds. Live poultry are normally imported as commercial breeding stock, and after a period in quarantine they or their progeny will be introduced directly into the main stream of the national poultry flock. There will be opportunity for close contact with the indigenous poultry through sharing sites or buildings, through common hatcheries and processing plants, and via vehicles, equipment and personnel.

Imported captive birds other than poultry are not likely to come into such direct contact with poultry. Certain diseases however, and particularly Newcastle disease, can spread by aerosol in the wind for considerable distances, and there have been serious outbreaks of Newcastle disease in poultry associated with the importation of captive birds.

The catastrophic epizootic of Newcastle disease that decimated the Californian poultry industry in 1971 was clearly linked to the importation of psittacine birds from South America. In this outbreak nine million birds were destroyed as part of a control programme that cost US$56 million (Lancaster & Alexander 1975). Imported tropical birds were also considered possible origins for the outbreaks of Newcastle disease in Holland (Roepke 1973) and England in 1970. In 1975 there was a link between three isolated and connected cases of Newcastle disease in poultry in southern England and an importation of sick psittacine birds from Southeast Asia.

IMPORTATIONS OF CARCASSES AND EGGS

Avian pathogens can also be transmitted in uncooked poultry carcasses and in eggs. Infected poultry meat fed to a small flock of poultry was almost certainly the way Newcastle disease came into England in 1926 (Doyle 1927). The outbreaks of this disease that occurred in the United Kingdom in 1947 were also linked to imports of poultry meat from Eastern Europe (Brown 1965). The bacterium *Salmonella pullorum* can spread from a parent flock via the egg to chicks by true transovarian vertical transmission. Probably all avian pathogens could enter the egg by mechanical means as it cools following surface contamination of the shell. If the embryo does not die, this can result in infection of the newly hatched chicks. Uncooked shells and shell membranes could be included in waste food and fed to chickens or other birds. Contamination of egg powder with salmonellae has also occurred and could be the source of human illness.

EXCLUSION OF AVIAN PATHOGENS

The simplest and surest way of excluding avian pathogens from a country is by completely banning the importation of any live bird, hatching egg or uncooked poultry product. In practice this is usually not a feasible proposition. Even if a country is self-sufficient in poultry products, it may need to import breeding stock to improve its genetic pool and productivity. Certain trading agreements between countries or groups of countries might also prevent total exclusion of imports of live poultry. It is also very difficult for a country to enforce a total ban on the importation of captive birds other than poultry. The demand for such birds as pets or for exhibition by people in Western Europe and North America seems insatiable (Ashton 1984). If too rigid a control policy is adopted, the price of birds increases and with it the likelihood of unsupervized illegal importation.

It must also be remembered that certain avian pathogens can be transported over considerable distances by migrating birds (Bourne, this volume).

Import controls for live birds

A country will try to prevent the introduction of avian pathogens with live birds by a system of import regulations. These vary from country to country and to a great extent are governed by the value and disease status of the national poultry flock in that locality. The importing country is entitled, subject to certain trading agreements, to impose what import conditions it requires. These vary considerably, from a basic requirement asking only that the birds have been inspected and found to be clinically healthy, to detailed and stringent criteria. There are, however, certain conditions in respect of poultry common to the import requirements of many countries and these will be outlined.

Poultry are usually imported as day-old chicks, and a usual request is for the parent flock to have been inspected and the birds found to be clinically healthy. The inspecting veterinary surgeon is usually asked to certify that the flock of origin has been free from certain diseases for a specified period of time. The import certificate is likely to stipulate that the flock of origin, or a percentage of that flock, has been blood-tested for certain diseases such as pullorum disease and mycoplasmosis with negative results. In addition, many countries require the flock of origin to be a member of a government supervized health scheme and an area clearance for Newcastle disease is usually mandatory. In the case of captive birds or poultry imported as growers or adults, the birds themselves would have to be inspected in the country of origin by an authorized veterinary surgeon and found to be healthy.

If the birds satisfy these criteria prior to import they would then be licensed into approved quarantine premises where they would remain for a number of weeks under close veterinary supervision. The quarantine premises would consist of secure buildings situated in an area free of indigenous poultry flocks. Any birds dying would be examined at an approved laboratory and a proportion of the carcasses checked for Newcastle disease virus.

Import controls on poultry products

Conditions can also be applied to the flocks of origin before a country will accept the import of poultry meat or eggs for eating. In the case of poultry meat these could require inspection of the birds, before slaughter, by an authorized veterinary surgeon. The birds would then have to be slaughtered in an approved processing plant, followed by veterinary inspection of the carcasses. Eggs for human consumption, and poultry meat, may also need to be accompanied by a certificate confirming that no Newcastle disease has occurred in the holding of origin or within a ten kilometre radius of these premises for at least six months.

ELIMINATION OF AVIAN PATHOGENS

It is easier to exclude an avian pathogen from a country than to eliminate it once it is established. In order to eliminate a disease it needs to be well defined, easily diagnosed or detectable by a simple, cheap and rapidly applied test (Hunter, this volume). A scheme for complete eradication of a disease from a country can be a massive operation requiring enormous financial and manpower resources. The history of attempts to eradicate Newcastle disease from the United Kingdom illustrates the difficulty of getting rid of a disease that can be present in a mild or subclinical form in a country with a large intensive poultry industry. The peracute form of the disease was effectively controlled by a slaughter policy between 1936 and 1947. When milder forms of the disease appeared in 1948, eradication by slaughter and compensation proved less effective. There were delays in reporting and diagnosing the mild and subacute forms of the disease. This coincided with a dramatic increase in the country's poultry population and in the adoption by the industry of intensive systems of management. In 1963 the slaughter policy was abandoned and replaced by a system of control by vaccination.

Two diseases which have been eliminated from commercial poultry flocks are *Salmonella pullorum* infection and mycoplasmosis. Many countries with a progressive poultry industry have eliminated pullorum disease from commercial flocks by a programme of blood-testing breeding flocks and culling reactors. Mycoplasmosis has also been controlled by either blood-testing or dipping hatching eggs into an antibiotic solution. Both these infections spread vertically from parent to progeny through the hatching egg and have a limited ability to spread laterally to other flocks in the vicinity. The difficulty of eliminating even infections such as these is illustrated by the fact that 30 years of continuous blood-testing was necessary to rid poultry breeding flocks of pullorum disease in the United Kingdom.

Chlamydia psittaci infection in a group of psittacine birds may take the form of severe clinical disease with heavy mortality but may also be subclinical, with carrier birds. It is possible to eliminate this infection from a group of infected birds by continuous feed medication with chlortetracycline for 45 days. This treatment regime has to be supported by a high standard of hygiene and management in the aviary. In some countries such a procedure is a mandatory requirement for all psittacine birds in quarantine.

CONTROL OF AVIAN PATHOGENS

Certain diseases may not lend themselves to elimination and eradication, but can be controlled effectively by vaccination and strategic medication. Viral infections such as Marek's disease, infectious bronchitis, infectious bursal disease and infectious laryngotracheitis can be well controlled by the correct use of vaccines now available. Chickens respond remarkably well to a wide range of live and inactivated vaccines. For example, one injection of a live Marek's disease vaccine to a day-old chick gives solid, long-lasting immunity that protects the bird for life.

Live vaccines are relatively inexpensive and have the advantage that they can usually be given in the water or by spray, thus allowing simple mass flock application. Inactivated vaccines have to be given to each bird by injection, but this ensures that each bird receives the full dose of vaccine. Such vaccines give a long-lasting high level of immunity, particularly if the bird has been primed with a live vaccine some weeks earlier. When such effective vaccines are available, control of an infectious disease by vaccination becomes more cost effective than eradication and elimination. Parasitic diseases such as coccidiosis and ascaridiasis can be controlled by strategic use of the coccidiostats and anthelmintics now available. Bacterial diseases, for example fowl cholera and tuberculosis, can be controlled by improved hygiene and modern management systems.

HEALTH STATUS OF IMPORTED BIRDS

Importations of commercial poultry for breeding are likely to be valuable healthy stock coming from a country with a sophisticated, high health-status poultry industry. Importations of non-domesticated species, however, come from any country, and in many cases the birds in question have been caught in the wild shortly before export. Sometimes they are accompanied by veterinary certification; sometimes not. The health of these birds is therefore an unknown quantity and they could carry with them a variety of avian pathogens. A survey of captive birds dying in quarantine was carried out at the Gloucester Veterinary Investigation Centre between 1975 and 1986 and involved 41 quarantine lots. These varied in size from 200 to 18,000 birds, and were usually made up of a variety of different species from a number of different sources. Most of the birds came directly from India, Taiwan, Senegal and Tanzania, but some came via dealers in Holland or Belgium. Seven different viruses were isolated from carcasses examined in the survey and these were Newcastle disease virus, paramyxovirus (PMV) 2 and 3, avian influenza viruses H3, H4 and H11, and a reovirus. Before 1979, influenza viruses were regularly isolated from the imported captive bird carcasses, but after 1979 no influenza viruses were isolated. Paramyxovirus 2 was most frequently isolated from non-psittacines, while paramyxovirus 3 was isolated only from members of the Psittaciformes. Reoviruses were isolated on five occasions from Grey Parrots (*Psittacus erithacus*) imported from Zaire, and were associated with necrosis of the liver and high mortality. *Chlamydia psittaci* was detected in most import lots that contained large numbers of psittacines. *Salmonella typhimurium* was frequently isolated from the carcasses of birds dying in quarantine but, surprisingly, other salmonella serotypes were not found. The phage types most frequently encountered were dt 93, 69, 80 and 49, but many isolates were untypable. On two occasions U286 was isolated from Grey Parrots imported from West Africa.

Tapeworm infestations were regularly found on examination of carcasses of small passerine birds. These parasites were invariably associated with high mortality and were difficult to treat. The tapeworms were identified as *Davainea*, *Raillietina* and *Cotugnia* species. Infection of small passerine birds with flagellate protozoa was also frequently encountered in the survey. The affected birds showed signs of respiratory distress, followed by heavy mortality. Necrotic lesions were found in the buccal mucosa and in the lining of the oesophagus and crop. Coccidiosis was never diagnosed in birds from any of the 41 quarantine lots examined.

APPLICATIONS TO THREATENED BIRD POPULATIONS

The precautions outlined above can be applied to threatened bird populations, whether free-living or captive. The exclusion of potential pathogens will depend largely on the restriction of movement of live birds, eggs or carcasses from elsewhere. Other items may also be potentially dangerous—for example, imported food (whether of animal or plant origin), semen, equipment used for catching free-living birds (e.g. bags and nets) or in the management of captive ones (e.g. incubators, brooders, gloves). Pests may be introduced inadvertently—for instance, rodents, cockroaches and mosquitoes. Little can be done to minimize the risk from migrating birds (Bourne, this volume) but the

Table 1: Exclusion of avian pathogens.

Source	Methods of exclusion
Birds and other live animals.	Careful screening and selection of incoming stock. Strict adherence to importation regulations where present. Quarantining (isolation) on arrival, coupled with appropriate tests. Exclusion and control of pests.
Animal products, e.g. carcasses, tissues, eggs, semen.	Careful screening and selection of incoming samples. Disinfection where feasible before despatch and on arrival. Strict adherence to importation regulations where present.
Inanimate material, e.g. equipment, clothing.	Careful screening and selection of incoming material. Disinfection or sterilization before despatch, on arrival, and at disposal.

careful siting of reserves and captive breeding programmes, or the construction of artificial pools so as to attract migrants away from the birds at risk, may go some way towards reducing the dangers. Ways in which the risk of introduction of pathogens from sources other than migrants may be minimized are summarized in *Table 1*.

If live birds are to be imported or brought into a locality in which a threatened species is at risk, various precautions are essential. Suggested guidelines are as follows:

1) Avoid bringing in birds unless, a) the importation is essential—for example, in order to increase the gene pool or to serve as foster birds, or b) the imports are known to be clinically healthy and free of potentially dangerous pathogens. Screening of birds is always wise (see Appendix 1), preferably at their place of origin before despatch.

It may even be wise to impose a total ban on the importation of certain species—for example, Greenwood & Cooper (1982) drew attention to the likely dangers presented by Prairie Falcons (*Falco mexicanus*) and Great-horned Owls (*Bubo virginianus*), both of which are commonly infected with falcon herpesvirus, and suggested that the importation of these species into Great Britain should be restricted or banned. Similar arguments have been put forward in the context of Mauritius where the Mauritius Kestrel (*Falco punctatus*) and Pink Pigeon (*Nesoenas mayeri*) populations might be put at risk if a herpesvirus (or perhaps a paramyxovirus) were introduced with imported birds (Cooper, Jones, this volume). Until recently the Australian government has maintained a total ban on the importation and exportation of non-domesticated birds. At the time of writing, this policy is being reviewed and the various consultation documents make interesting and useful reading for those who are concerned with disease control.

2) If birds are to be brought in they must be quarantined (isolated) for a minimum of five weeks, during which time they can be observed, examined clinically and screened for pathogens. If clinical disease or deaths occur the quarantine should be extended for at least two more weeks.

The use of clean 'sentinel' birds which can be monitored and examined (live or dead) has much to commend it. Sentinel fowl are regularly used in quarantine stations in Britain, and a number of other species have been employed in attempts to detect pathogens in free-living birds—for example, sentinel ducks and turkeys in work on avian paramyxoviruses (Kelleher *et al.* 1985).

Tests than can be carried out on birds in quarantine, including sentinels, are outlined by Hunter (this volume). Strict adherence to quarantine rules is essential, as is the implementation of high standards of hygiene. Various disinfectants can be used to minimize the spread of infection: examples are given by Cooper (1986), who also provided information on how the ability of birds to resist infection and disease might best be enhanced.

Although live birds probably represent the greatest threat, the danger of introducing pathogens with other animals (e.g. rodents brought in as food for raptors), carcasses, tissues, biological samples and inanimate objects must not be underestimated. In some countries, Government restrictions designed to protect the health of humans or domestic animals help to ensure that potentially hazardous organisms are not imported (M. E. Cooper, this volume) but this may not be the case in countries where threatened birds are often most at risk.

Once a pathogen has entered a population a decision has to be made whether to attempt to eliminate it, to control it or to take no action whatsoever. The course to be followed depends on a number of factors. As a general rule the only pathogens that warrant action (elimination or control) are those that are likely either a) to cause a high mortality, or b) to reduce reproductive performance in the birds at risk. However, the cost, in terms of time and money, of implementing an elimination or control programme has to be considered. Some diseases are easily diagnosed or the causal organisms detected in the live or dead bird, in which case control can be attempted by means of such measures as isolation/culling of affected individuals, vaccination, chemotherapy or a combination of all three. Other disease organisms may be more difficult to detect and more insidious in their effects. These may well defy attempts to eliminate or control them. An understanding of the biology of different disease-causing organisms is needed if a correct decision is to be made (Reece, this volume).

The success or otherwise of a particular control measure will depend on a number of factors. Particularly important is the rate at which the introduced pathogen is spreading and its ability to persist both within the host species and outside (for example, in arthropod vectors, in water or soil, in nestboxes or as airborne particles). These in turn will be influenced by the numbers and density of avian hosts and the interaction between the pathogen and predators/competitors. The advice of epidemiologists and statisticians can prove valuable in analysing the situation.

There are other ways in which the effects of pathogens on threatened birds can be minimized. If birds are healthy, clinical disease is probably less likely to be a problem but the fact that many avian populations are isolated and often have had no previous exposure to certain pathogens may make them particularly vulnerable. In due course breeding for disease resistance, perhaps by genetic manipulation, as suggested in the fowl (Freeman & Bumstead 1987) may be desirable.

CONCLUSIONS

Threatened birds are at risk from pathogens from many quarters. The chances of organisms establishing themselves and spreading will be minimized if basic precautions are followed. Much can be learned from the experiences of those who for many years have been involved in excluding diseases from poultry flocks or eliminating/controlling them once they have become established. Disease control is a complex subject: it could and should involve people from many different disciplines.

REFERENCES

ASHTON, W. L. G. 1984. The risks and problems connected with the import and export of captive birds. *Br. Vet. J.* **140**: 317–27.
BROWN, A. C. L. 1965. The epidemiology of Newcastle disease in Great Britain. *Proc. Roy. Soc. Med.* **58**: 801–2.
COOPER, J. E. 1986. Preventive medicine in birds of prey. *In:* Fowler, M. E. (ed.). *Zoo and Wild Animal Medicine*, 2nd edition. W. B. Saunders, Philadelphia.
DOYLE, T. M. 1927. A hitherto unrecorded disease of fowls due to a filter passing virus. *J. Comp. Path. Ther.* **40**: 144–69.
FREEMAN, B. M. & BUMSTEAD, N. 1987. Breeding for disease resistance—the prospective role of genetic manipulation. *Avian Path.* **16**: 353–65.
GREENWOOD, A. G. & COOPER, J. E. 1982. Herpesvirus infections in falcons. *Vet. Rec.* **111**: 514.
KELLEHER, C. J., HALVORSON, D. A., NEWMAN, J. A. & SENNE, D. A. 1985. Isolation of avian paramyxoviruses from sentinel ducks and turkeys in Minnesota. *Avian Dis.* **29**: 400–07.
LANCASTER, J. E. & ALEXANDER, D. J. 1975. Newcastle disease virus and spread. *Monograph No. 11.* Canada Department of Agriculture.
ROEPKE, W. J. 1973. The control of Newcastle disease in the Netherlands. *Proceedings of 4th European Poultry Conference*, London.

MICROBIOLOGICAL INVESTIGATION OF WILD BIRDS

F. T. SCULLION

Department of Pathology, University of Bristol, School of Veterinary Science, Comparative Pathology Laboratory, Langford House, Langford, Bristol BS18 7DU, England

ABSTRACT

This paper outlines the correct procedures for submitting samples to a laboratory for microbiological investigation, and introduces the methods employed in the identification of various groups of micro-organisms. The clinical significance of microbiological results is discussed with the aid of tables of some of the diseases in wild birds associated with various organisms.

INTRODUCTION

Disease investigation requires an ability to correlate information obtained from a history, physical examination, post-mortem findings and relevant laboratory data. Microbiology, a laboratory-based study of organisms not visible to the naked eye, has evolved around the investigation of disease. However, due to their ubiquitous nature and the fact that most microbes are non-pathogenic, results from laboratory tests are not a panacea for all diagnostic problems. Instead they should be considered one of many aids to diagnosis. The true value of microbiology in disease investigation can only be fully appreciated with an understanding of the basic principles of the science.

SUBMISSION OF SAMPLES TO A LABORATORY

The value of laboratory results is always improved with adequate preparation and proper selection, handling, and transportation of specimens.

Preparation
A microbiological laboratory will attempt to isolate and identify all significant organisms in submitted samples. To be effective, most laboratories employ routine procedures which allow them to attain this standard as often as possible. Since some classes of microbes can be isolated only with the aid of specialized facilities, it is advisable to check before submitting samples to establish if the laboratory's procedures are adequate for the isolation of the particular microbes

that are considered important in the case under investigation. Advice will be given on their preferred methods of handling, packaging and transportation of samples.

Selection of specimens

The type of sample submitted can have a bearing on the reliability of the results obtained. Specimens can be taken from either live or dead birds.

Live birds: Ideally, samples for bacterial or viral isolation from live birds should be collected in the early stages of the disease process before treatment has commenced. There are relatively few sites in the live bird from which samples can be obtained without contamination precluding accurate representation and it is necessary to consider these facts when interpreting results. Isolates from the cloaca will reflect the microbial flora not only of the distal bowel but also, possibly, of the urinary and reproductive tracts. Crop samples obtained by a sterile saline wash can become contaminated with flora from the upper digestive tract (Drewes & Flammer 1986). Swabs from the choanal orifice may be representative of the respiratory tract but again there is danger of contamination from the upper digestive tract. Nasal swabs are generally considered to be contaminated with external flora (Richter & Gerlach 1981).

In live birds it is possible to culture blood samples obtained using aseptic techniques (Kollias *et al.* 1987) and with various surgical procedures representative samples can be obtained from sites such as the air sacs, sinuses, crop, liver and other internal organs which may prove to be more useful in determining the aetiological significance of various isolates in disease investigations (Harrison & Harrison 1986).

Dead birds: In the dead bird, lesions can be swabbed directly or pieces of tissue can be submitted for examination. Necropsy procedures should ensure that samples are not overly contaminated (Harrigan 1981). One major disadvantage of using material from dead birds is that any delay in performing the post-mortem examination allows the invasion of microbes throughout the body. Enteric bacteria are frequently isolated from internal organs following such delays, and this leads to difficulty in the interpretation of findings. Carcasses should therefore be refrigerated at 4°C if a post-mortem examination cannot be carried out immediately.

Handling and transportation of specimens

Swabs are convenient for taking samples from a lesion but unfortunately they only suffice for small sample volumes. Delay in transferring the sample to a culture plate can result in desiccation, and the death of many of the microbes present. This can be avoided by using commercial swabs such as 'Transwab' and 'Transwab E.N.T.' (Medical Wire and Equipment Co. Ltd., Polley, Corsham, Wilts., England), which incorporate a sterile transport medium. Milk saline swabs can be obtained by request from the laboratory for the submission of samples for virus isolation. Some microbes require particular transport media and for some others certain types of swabs may be deleterious.

Normally, to preserve bacteria and prevent deterioration, specimens can be refrigerated to 4°C before transportation. Bearing in mind postal regulations (M. E. Cooper, this volume), packages for transportation should be secured so that they will not leak and damage other mail or cause a health hazard. Samples for virus isolation should be frozen and packed in ice (wet or dry) with the refrigerant making up 50 percent of the weight of the package. They should be placed in leak-proof plastic, surrounded by absorbent material and protected from damage by an outer covering of wood or sturdy cardboard. Alternatively, the laboratory selected to examine the specimen for viruses can give advice on transportation of samples if ice is not available. The outside of the container should be labelled 'Biological Specimen' or 'Pathological Specimen' and 'Fragile with Care' but the exact wording will depend on the postal regulations of the country involved. The inclusion of a detailed relevant history with the clinical and post-mortem examination findings is always greatly appreciated. For some viruses, such as herpesviruses, chilled specimens or specimens on dry ice are of more value than frozen specimens, which emphasizes the need to have some idea of the likely isolate.

METHODS EMPLOYED IN IDENTIFYING VARIOUS GROUPS OF MICRO-ORGANISMS

The major groups of microbes that are particularly relevant to any discussion on microbiological investigation in wild birds are bacteria, viruses and fungi. The nomenclature and systems of classification adhered to in this discussion are similar to those found in Bergey's *Manual of Systematic Bacteriology* (Holt 1986) for bacteria, *Classification and Nomenclature of Viruses* (Matthews 1979) for viruses, and *Essentials of Veterinary Bacteriology and Mycology* (Carter 1976) for fungi.

Microbes are isolated and propagated in the laboratory as a pure culture, and characteristics diagnostic for particular groups are used in identification (Hitchner *et al.* 1980).

Bacteria

Bacteria can be primarily classified by their staining characteristics and morphology.

A differential stain such as Gram's stain can divide bacteria into two groups, Gram-positives and Gram-negatives, and thus it is possible to note the Gram staining reaction, size and shape of the bacteria, whether or not they contain endospores and if so their size, shape and intracellular position, and so derive a tentative classification. Another differential stain, Ziehl-Neelsen, is especially useful in demonstrating *Mycobacterium* or *Nocardia* species.

In all cases, however, cultural procedures are necessary to arrive at a specific identification. When bacteria are grown on a solid laboratory medium, such as fresh blood agar, the size, colour, translucency and shape of the colonies are criteria used in the identification process. Certain bacteria also have additional characteristic growth requirements in the laboratory. For example, the bacterial requirements for oxygen have led to three distinct groupings of aerobic, anaerobic and facultative anaerobic organisms being recognized.

Special culture media may also be used to identify bacteria. Selective media contain substances that inhibit all but a few types of organism. Indicator media contain sugars such as glucose, lactose, and mannitol which certain bacteria will ferment, resulting in the production of acid which creates a colour change in indicators contained in the media. Other special media can indicate end-products of biochemical reactions, such as the generation of hydrogen sulphide gas or whether the bacteria contain enzymes such as urease, gelatinase etc. For example, biselenite broth is a selective medium used to culture *Salmonella* species, and is particularly useful when investigating possible carrier birds. MacConkey agar is an indicator medium used to differentiate lactose- and non-lactose-fermenting enteric bacteria.

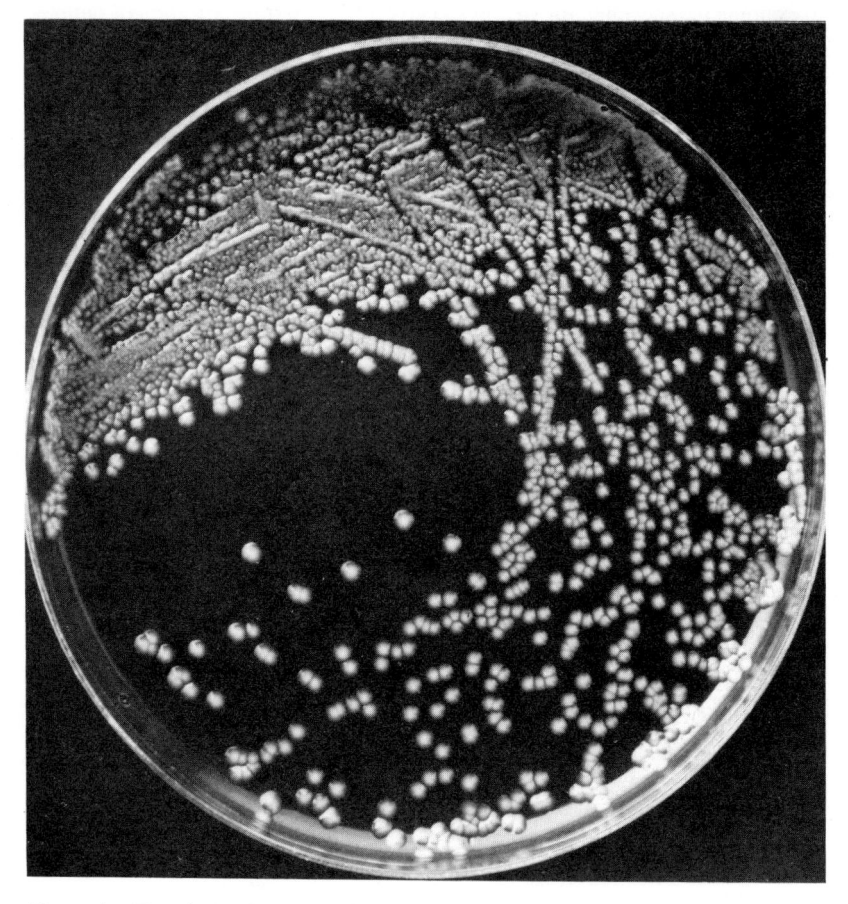

Figure 1: The size, colour, translucency and shape of colonies are criteria used in identifying bacteria. (*Photo:* Scullion)

Specific antisera can be valuable in serotyping bacteria and use is also made of a group of viruses, called bacteriophages, which cause lysis of bacteria, to biotype individual strains.

Animal pathogenicity or toxicity tests are also sometimes used to identify bacteria. The only reliable test to identify the toxin produced by the bacterium *Clostridium botulinum*, which causes botulism (Reece, this volume), involves animal inoculation.

Antibiotic sensitivity testing, although mostly used as a guide to the choice of antibiotics for therapy, can also be used as an epidemiological marker in some studies.

Viruses

Many viruses have been implicated in diseases of birds on the basis of histopathological and electron-microscopic examination of lesions. Much work

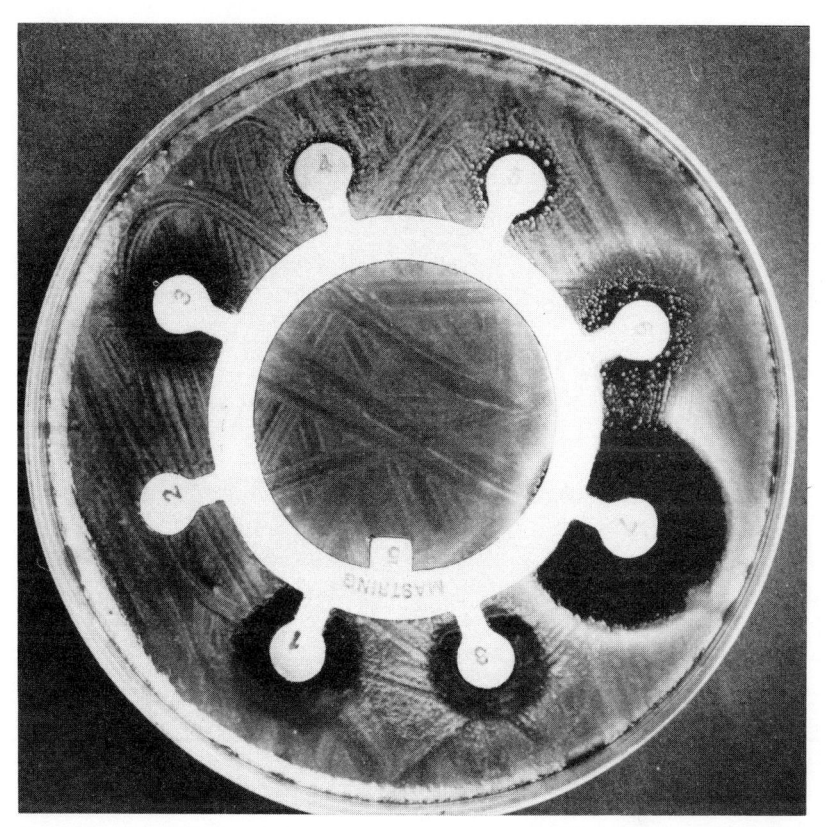

Figure 2: Antibiotic sensitivity testing may be used as an epidemiological marker and as an aid to treatment of affected birds. (*Photo:* Scullion)

needs to be done, however, in terms of the isolation and identification of viruses before their full role in avian diseases is determined. The isolation and propagation of viruses require specialized techniques (Versteeg 1985). Viruses can be cultivated only in living cells, and although some can grow in a wide range of cell systems others will multiply only in a narrow range of natural host cells. A number of viruses require a few serial passages before they are identifiable in the laboratory culture system. The most frequently used cell systems for avian viruses are tissue and organ cultures, and occasionally chick embryos or live animals may be used. It should be noted that there are very few established avian cell lines available for routine work, which is in contradistinction to the many available mammalian cell lines. Therefore most avian tissue culture involves killing a bird to harvest various organs and tissues.

Viral cytopathogenic effects in cell cultures or chick embryos, which are visible grossly or microscopically, along with other characteristics such as route of inoculation, incubation time, temperature etc., can be valuable in identification. Methods involved in further differentiation may include haemagglutination of red blood cells from various species of animals, haemadsorption of red blood cells to infected cells in the culture system, or investigation of biochemical,

Table 1: Bacteria associated with disease in wild birds.

Genus	Laboratory characteristics (Cottral 1978)	Associated clinical signs/disease	Susceptibility	References
Staphylococcus	Aerobic, facultatively anaerobic Gram-positive cocci, grow in irregular grape-like clusters on blood agar. Form acid from glucose; produce catalase.	Septicaemia; arthritis; osteitis; bumblefoot	Anseriformes; Columbiformes; Falconiformes; Galliformes; Passeriformes; Piciformes	Cooper 1987; Jennings 1954; Keymer 1958A; Keymer 1958B
Streptococcus	Aerobic, Gram-positive cocci; chain-forming; Septicaemia pinhead-size colonies on blood agar. Produce acid on carbohydrate media.		Psittaciformes; Passeriformes	Schultz 1981
Erysipelothrix	Aerobic, facultatively anaerobic Gram-positive slender hair-like bacilli. Tiny smooth colonies on culture.	Septicaemia	Anseriformes; Charadriiformes; Ciconiformes; Columbiformes; Galliformes; Gaviformes; Gruiformes; Passeriformes; Podicipediformes; Strigiformes	Blackmore & Gallagher 1964; Decker et al. 1977; Bach et al. 1987
Listeria	Aerobic, Gram-positive rods. Occur in pairs—may resemble diplococci. Form 1–2mm grey translucent colonies on culture; clear zones of haemolysis on blood agar. Grow in 10% NaCl.	Septicaemia; encephalitis, chronic wasting	Anseriformes; Charadriiformes; Columbiformes; Falconiformes; Galliformes; Passeriformes; Psittaciformes; Strigiformes	Fowler 1986; Wallach & Boever 1983
Clostridium	Anaerobic, Gram-positive spore-bearing rods; spores resistant to environmental conditions. C. botulinum produces toxin; spores develop when environmental temperature rises.	Fatal toxicity (e.g. botulism)	Anseriformes; Ciconiformes; Columbiformes; Coraciformes; Galliformes; Gruiformes; Passeriformes; Piciformes	Cambre 1987; Reece, this volume
Escherichia*	Aerobic, Gram-negative rods. Produce pink colonies on MacConkey agar.	Septicaemia; enteritis; respiratory disease; reproductive tract disease; generalized granulomatous infection	Anseriformes; Galliformes; Falconiformes; Passeriformes; Psittaciformes; Sphenisciformes	Fowler 1986

Salmonella*	Aerobic, Gram-negative rods. Produce grey colonies on MacConkey agar.	Enteritis; carrier state; septicaemia	Charadriiformes; Columbiformes; Gaviiformes; Passeriformes; Pelicaniformes; Sphenisciformes	Faddoul et al. 1966; Oelke & Steiniger 1973; White et al. 1976; Wilson & Macdonald 1967
Shigella*	Aerobic, Gram-negative rods. Produce grey or colourless colonies on MacConkey agar.	Enteritis	Anseriformes	Fiennes 1982
Pasteurella*	Aerobic, Gram-negative non motile ovoid rods.	Respiratory disease; new duck disease; goose influenza; septicaemia	Anseriformes; Galliformes; Passeriformes	Faddoul et al. 1967; Davis et al. 1971
Yersinia*	Aerobic, Gram-negative rods.	Generalised granulomatous infection; sudden death; wasting disease	Coraciiformes; Falconiformes; Musophagiformes; Passeriformes; Piciformes; Psittaciformes	Obwolo 1976
Haemophilus	Aerobic, Gram-negative coccobacilli. Grow on chocolate agar; some strains require 10% CO_2.	Respiratory disease; sinusitis	Galliformes	Wallach & Boever 1983
Mycobacterium	Ziehl-Neelsen positive; require specialized techniques for isolation and identification.	Generalized tubercular lesions; enteric spread in birds—usually Mycobacterium avium. Diffuse granulomatous thickening in some species	All orders thought susceptible	Montali et al. 1976; Forster & Gerlach 1987
Mycoplasma	Aerobic; some require 10% CO_2; pleomorphic bacteria with no cell wall; need specialized techniques for isolation and identification.	Respiratory disease; conjunctivitis; sinusitis	Falconiformes; Passeriformes; Psittaciformes	Gaskin 1987; Furr et al. 1977
Chlamydia	Require living cells for isolation; many strains with varying pathogenicity.	Psittacosis; ornithosis; chlamydiosis; respiratory disease; enteritis; carrier state; conjunctivitis	All Orders thought susceptible, but especially the Psittaciformes and Columbiformes which may be silently infected	Johnson 1983; Reece (this volume)

Note: *Biochemical, serological and phage typing tests are used to differentiate various Gram-negative organisms and to identify the species and strains.

serological and electron-microscopic properties. Of these, serological identification provides the backbone of most virus identification systems.

More recently, molecular biological techniques have been developed that can accurately identify specific regions of viral nucleic acid in infected tissues as well as identify the nucleic acid in virus cultured from clinical samples in the laboratory (Herring & Sharp 1984), though such sophisticated techniques are not in common use for avian viruses.

Fungi
Fungi are relatively easy to culture in the laboratory on special media that contain antibacterials to prevent interference by other microbes. Due to the much slower growth characteristics of most fungi the identification procedures are delayed, and as a corollary of this, fungal diseases in animals tend to be slowly progressive. Fungal identification is based on the morphological characteristics of various stages of the fungal life-cycle with or without additional biochemical tests (Ainsworth & Austwick 1973; Evans & Gentles 1985).

CLINICAL SIGNIFICANCE OF FINDINGS

Much of what is known about the diseases of birds is derived from studies on diseases of man and domestic animals including the domestic chicken. There are a number of texts dealing with diseases of captive wild mammals and birds (Davis et al. 1971; Petrak 1982; Wallach & Boever 1983; Fowler 1986; Harrison & Harrison 1986). Unfortunately, in this fledgling branch of medicine much of the scientific evidence for the role of microbes in diseases of wild birds is based on descriptive studies and comparative medical deductive and inductive reasoning. Descriptive studies have a number of inherent defects when used to interpret causation (Dohoo & Waltner-Toews 1985). It is important, therefore, that investigators continually strive to improve the science of wildlife medicine by critical analysis of current knowledge and the use of carefully designed studies that will either substantiate or refute present theories. Some of the following information on microbial diseases of wild birds is based on single case reports so it is obvious that much work is needed in this particular field before general statements can be made with certainty.

MICROBES ASSOCIATED WITH DISEASES IN BIRDS

Tables 1, 2 and *3* list the major groups of bacteria, viruses and fungi respectively that have been associated with disease in wild birds. Orders of susceptible birds are listed to help illustrate the universal nature of many disease processes but the lists should by no means be considered complete. Inevitably, any attempt to summarize such a vast amount of information in tabular form will be tainted with the brush of oversimplification. However, it is hoped that the inclusion of these tables will have the opposite effect and that the reader will realize the boundless task that lies ahead of the scientist interested in this field of endeavour. References are provided to stimulate further indulgence.

Table 2: Viruses associated with disease in wild birds.

Virus group	Associated disease/clinical signs	Major organ system affected	Susceptibility	References
Adenoviruses	Budgerigar adenovirus	Liver; pancreas	Psittaciformes	Lowenstine 1986
	Quail bronchitis	Respiratory	Galliformes	Wallach & Boever 1983
Herpesviruses	Pacheco's disease	Liver	Psittaciformes	Ashton 1988
	Duck plague	Intestine	Anseriformes	Gough 1984
	Falcon herpes	Liver	Falconiformes	Gerlach 1986
	Owl herpes	Liver	Strigiformes	Gerlach 1986
	Amazon tracheitis	Respiratory	Psittaciformes	Gerlach 1986
	Herpes ciconiae	Liver	Ciconiiformes	Gerlach 1986
	Crane herpes	Liver	Gruiformes	Docherty & Henning 1980
	Marek's disease	Nervous	Falconiformes; Strigiformes	Keymer 1972 Halliwell 1971
Orbiviruses (Reoviridae)	Hepatic necrosis	Liver	Psittaciformes	Graham 1987
Papovaviruses	Sudden death	Liver	Psittaciformes	Graham & Calnek 1987
	Sudden death	Generalized infection	Passeriformes	Forshaw et al. 1988
	Papillomas	Intestine	Psittaciformes	Lowenstine 1986
Myxoviruses	Newcastle disease (fowl pest)	Central nervous system; respiratory; intestine	All Orders thought susceptible	Beard & Hanson 1984 Bourne (this volume)
	Influenza virus (fowl plague)	Central nervous system	Columbiformes	Alexander et al. 1984
	Pigeon paramyxovirus	Central nervous system	Psittaciformes	Mannl et al. 1987
	Wasting macaw syndrome			
Parvoviruses	Goose virus hepatitis	Liver	Anseriformes	Schettler 1971
Parvo-like viruses	Psittacine beak and feather syndrome	Integument	Psittaciformes	Wylie & Pass 1987 McOrist (this volume)
Picornaviruses	Duck virus hepatitis	Liver	Anseriformes	Sandhu 1986
Poxviruses	Avian pox	Integument	All Orders thought susceptible	Gerlach 1986 Jenkins et al. (this volume)
Togaviruses	Eastern equine encephalitis virus infection	Non specific illness; carrier state	Anseriformes; Ciconiiformes; Columbiformes; Galliformes; Gruiformes; Passeriformes	Ritchie 1987 Carpenter et al. (this volume)
Unclassified viruses	Puffinosis	Integument	Charadriiformes; Sphenisciformes	Stoskopf & Kennedy-Stoskopf 1986

Table 3: Fungi associated with disease in wild birds.

Fungus	Associated disease	Susceptibility	References
Aspergillus	Aspergillosis	All Orders thought susceptible	Wallach & Boever 1983
Candida	Candidiasis	All Orders thought susceptible	O'Meara & Witter 1971; Wallach & Boever 1983 Cooper 1978; Ainsworth & Austwick 1973

ACKNOWLEDGEMENTS

I would like to thank Dr Leighton Greenham for his comments on the manuscript and Miss A. McSorley for typing assistance.

REFERENCES

AINSWORTH, G. C. & AUSTWICK, P. K. C. 1973. *Fungal Diseases of Animals*. 2nd edition. Commonwealth Agricultural Bureaux, Farnham Royal, Slough.

ALEXANDER, D. J., WILSON, G. W. C., THAIN, J. A. & LISTER, S. A. 1984. Avian paramyxovirus type 1 infection of racing pigeons: III Epizootiological considerations. *Vet. Rec.* **115**: 213–16.

ASHTON, W. L. G. 1988. Pacheco's parrot disease and reovirus associated hepatitis. *In:* Price, C. J. (ed.) *Manual of Parrots Budgerigars and Other Psittacine Birds*. British Small Animal Veterinary Association, Cheltenham.

BACH, F., WACKER, R. & MAYER, H. 1987. Prophylaxis and therapy for erysipelas in marabou and other zoo birds. *Verh. ber. Erkrg. Zootiere.* **29**: 101–6.

BEARD, C. W. & HANSON, R. P. 1984. Newcastle disease. *In:* Hofstad, M. S., Barnes, H. J., Calnek, B. W., Reid, W. M. & Yoder, H. W. (eds) *Diseases of Poultry*. 8th edition. Iowa State University Press, Ames.

BLACKMORE, D. K. & GALLAGHER, G. L. 1964. An outbreak of erysipelas in captive wild birds and mammals. *Vet. Rec.* **76**: 1161–4.

CAMBRE, R. C. 1987. Avian botulism in a zoological garden—report of a two year outbreak. *Verh. ber. Erkrg. Zootiere* **29**: 19–24.

CARTER, G. R. 1976. *Essentials of Veterinary Bacteriology and Mycology*. Michigan State University Press, East Lansing.

COOPER, J. E. 1978. *Veterinary Aspects of Captive Birds of Prey*. Standfast Press, Saul, Gloucestershire.

COOPER, J. E. 1987. Pathological studies on avian pododermatitis (bumblefoot). *Verh. ber. Erkrg. Zootiere.* **29**: 107–14.

COTTRAL, G. E. 1978. *Manual of Standardised Methods for Veterinary Microbiology*. Cornell University Press, Ithaca.

DAVIS, J. W., ANDERSON, R. C., KARSTAD, L. & TRAINER, D. O. 1971. *Infectious and Parasitic Diseases of Wild Birds*. Iowa State University Press, Ames.

DECKER, R. A., LINDAUER, R. & ARCHIBALD, G. W. 1977. Erysipelothrix infection in two East African crowned cranes (*Balearica regulorum—gibbinceps*) and a wood duck (*Aix sponsa*). *Avian Dis.* **21**: 326–7.

DOCHERTY, D. E. & HENNING, D. J. 1980. The isolation of a herpesvirus from captive cranes with an inclusion body disease. *Avian Dis.* **24**: 278–83.

DOHOO, I. R. & WALTNER-TOEWS, D. W. 1985. Interpreting clinical research part II. Descriptive and experimental studies. *Compendium on Continuing Education for the Practicing Veterinarian.* **7**: S513–S520.

DREWES, L. A. & FLAMMER, K. 1986. Clinical microbiology. *In:* Harrison, G. J. &

Harrison, L. R. (eds). *Clinical Avian Medicine and Surgery.* W. B. Saunders Company, Philadelphia.
EVANS, E. G. V. & GENTLES, J. C. 1985. *Essentials of Medical Mycology.* Churchill Livingstone, Edinburgh.
FADDOUL, G. P., FELLOWS, G. W. & BAIRD, J. 1966. A survey on the incidence of salmonellae in wild birds. *Avian Dis.* **10**: 89–94.
FADDOUL, G. P., FELLOWS, G. W. & BAIRD, J. 1967. Pasteurellosis in wild birds in Massachusetts. *Avian Dis.* **11**: 413–18.
FIENNES, R. N. T-W. 1982. Diseases of bacterial origin. *In:* Petrak, M. L. (ed.). *Diseases of Cage and Aviary Birds.* 2nd edition. 497–515. Lea & Febiger, Philadelphia.
FORSHAW, D., WYLIE, S. L. & PASS, D. A. 1988. Infection with a virus resembling Papovavirus in Gouldian finches (*Erythrura gouldiae*). *Aust. Vet. J.* **65**: 26–8.
FORSTER, F. & GERLACH, H. 1987. Mycobacteria in Psittaciformes. *Proceedings of First International Conference on Zoological and Avian Medicine.* Omnipress, Madison, Wisconsin.
FOWLER, M. E. 1986. *Zoo and Wild Animal Medicine.* 2nd edition. W. B. Saunders Company, Philadelphia.
FURR, P. M., COOPER, J. E. & TAYLOR-ROBINSON, D. 1977. Isolation of mycoplasmas from three falcons (*Falco* spp.). *Vet. Rec.* **100**: 72–3.
GASKIN, J. N. 1987. Mycoplasmosis of caged birds. *In: Proceedings First International Conference on Zoological and Avian Medicine.* Omnipress, Madison, Wisconsin.
GERLACH, H. 1986. Viral diseases. *In:* Harrison, G. J. & Harrison, L. R. (eds). *Clinical Avian Medicine and Surgery.* W. B. Saunders Company, Philadelphia.
GOUGH, R. E. 1984. Laboratory confirmed outbreaks of duck virus enteritis (duck plague) in the United Kingdom from 1977 to 1982. *Vet. Rec.* **114**: 262–5.
GRAHAM, D. L. 1987. Characterization of a Reo-like virus and its isolation from and pathogenicity for parrots. *Avian Dis.* **31**: 411–19.
GRAHAM, D. L. & CALNEK, B. W. 1987. Papovavirus infection in hand fed parrots: virus isolation and pathology. *Avian Dis.* **31**: 398–410.
HALLIWELL, W. H. 1971. Lesions of Marek's disease in a Great Horned Owl. *Avian Dis.* **15**: 49–55.
HARRIGAN, K. E. 1981. Coping with and caring for dead birds—post mortems. *In: Aviary and Caged Birds.* Proceedings No. 55. The Post-Graduate Committee in Veterinary Science, The University of Sydney.
HARRISON, G. J. & HARRISON, L. R. 1986. *Clinical Avian Medicine and Surgery.* W. B. Saunders Company, Philadelphia.
HERRING, A. J. & SHARP, J. M. 1984. Protein blotting: The basic method and its role in viral diagnosis. *In:* McNulty, M. S. & McFerran, J. B. (eds). *Recent Advances in Virus Diagnosis.* Martinus Nijhoff Publishers, Boston.
HITCHNER, S. B., DOMERMUTH, C. H., PURCHASE, H. G. & WILLIAMS, J. E. 1980. *Isolation and Identification of Avian Pathogens.* 2nd edition. Am. Assoc. Avian Pathologists, Philadelphia.
HOLT, J. G. 1986. *Bergey's Manual of Systematic Bacteriology.* (Volumes 1 and 2.) Williams and Wilkins, Baltimore.
JENNINGS, A. R. 1954. Diseases in wild birds. *J. Comp. Path.* **64**: 356–9.
JOHNSON, F. W. A. 1983. Chlamydiosis. *Br. vet. J.* **139**: 93–101.
KEYMER, I. F. 1958A. A survey and review of the causes of mortality in British birds and the significance of wild birds as disseminators of disease—Part I. *Vet. Rec.* **70**: 713–20.
KEYMER, I. F. 1958B. A survey and review of the causes of mortality in British birds and the significance of wild birds as disseminators of disease—Part II. *Vet. Rec.* **70**: 736–40.
KEYMER, I. F. 1972. Diseases of birds of prey. *Vet. Rec.* **90**: 579–94.
KOLLIAS, G. V., HEARD, D. J., MARTIN, H. & COBURN, G. G. 1987. Principles, techniques and clinical use of blood cultures in birds. *Proceedings First International Conference on Zoological and Avian Medicine.* Omnipress, Madison, Wisconsin.
LOWENSTINE, L. J. 1986. Emerging viral diseases of psittacine birds. *In:* Kirk, R. W. (ed.). *Current Veterinary Therapy IX. Small Animal Practice.* W. B. Saunders Company, Philadelphia.

MANNL, A., GERLACH, H. & LEIPOLD, R. 1987. Neuropathic gastric dilation in psittaciformes. *Avian Dis.* **31**: 214–21.

MATTHEWS, R. E. F. 1979. *Classification and Nomenclature of Viruses; Third Report Prepared by the International Committee on Taxonomy of Viruses.* S. Karger, Basel.

MONTALI, R. J., BUSH, M., THOEN, C. O. & SMITH, E. 1976. Tuberculosis in captive exotic birds. *J. Am. vet. med. Ass.* **169**: 920–7.

OBWOLO, M. 1976. Yersiniosis in the Bristol Zoo 1955–1974. *Acta Zoologica et Pathologica Antverpiensia.* **64**: 81–90.

OELKE, H. & STEINIGER, F. 1973. Salmonella in Adelie Penguins (*Pygoscelis adeliae*) and South Polar Skuas (*Catharacta maccormicki*) on Ross Island, Antarctica. *Avian Dis.* **17**: 568–73.

O'MEARA, D. C. & WITTER, J. F. 1971. Candidiasis. *In:* Davis, J. W., Anderson, R. C., Karstad, L., & Trainer, D. O. (eds). *Infectious and Parasitic Diseases of Wild Birds.* Iowa State University Press, Ames.

PETRAK, M. L. 1982. *Diseases of Cage and Aviary Birds.* 2nd edition. Lea and Febiger, Philadelphia.

RICHTER, Th. & GERLACH, H. 1981. The bacterial flora of the nasal mucosa of birds of prey. *In:* Cooper, J. E. & Greenwood, A. G. (eds). *Recent Advances in the Study of Raptor Diseases.* Chiron Publications, Keighley.

RITCHIE, B. W. 1987. A review of eastern equine encephalomyelitis in pheasants. *AAV Today.* **1**(4): 152–4.

SANDHU, T. 1986. Duck virus hepatitis. *In:* Fowler, M. E. (ed.), *Zoo and Wild Animal Medicine.* 2nd edition. W. B. Saunders Company, Philadelphia.

SCHETTLER, C. H. 1971. Isolation of a highly pathogenic virus from geese with hepatitis. *Avian Dis.* **15**: 323–5.

SCHULTZ, D. J. 1981. Septicaemia: Aetiology, diagnosis and therapy. *In: Aviary and Caged Birds.* Proceedings No. 55. The Post-Graduate Committee in Veterinary Science, The University of Sydney.

STOSKOPF, M. K. & KENNEDY-STOSKOPF, S. 1986. Aquatic birds. *In:* Fowler, M. E. (ed.). *Zoo and Wild Animal Medicine.* 2nd edition. W. B. Saunders Company, Philadelphia.

VERSTEEG, J. 1985. *A Colour Atlas of Virology.* Wolfe Medical Publications, London.

WALLACH, J. D. & BOEVER, W. J. 1983. *Diseases of Exotic Animals.* W. B. Saunders Company, Philadelphia.

WHITE, F. H., FORRESTER, D. J. & NESBITT, S. I. 1976. Salmonella and Aspergillus infections in common loons overwintering in Florida. *J. Am. vet. med. Ass.* **169**(9): 936–7.

WILSON, J. E. & MACDONALD, A. W. 1967. Salmonella infection in wild birds. *Br. vet. J.* **123**: 212–19.

WYLIE, S. L. & PASS, D. A. 1987. Experimental reproduction of psittacine beak and feather disease/French moult. *Avian Path.* **16**: 269–81.

THE ROLE OF PATHOGENS IN THREATENED POPULATIONS: AN HISTORICAL REVIEW

J. E. COOPER

Department of Pathology, Royal College of Surgeons of England, 35–43 Lincoln's Inn Fields, London WC2A 3PN, England.

ABSTRACT

Micro-organisms and parasites can cause disease in both domesticated and wild birds, and often have a profound effect on captive populations. The impact of disease on free-living birds is less clear-cut but there is increasing evidence that it can cause significant morbidity and mortality, especially in small isolated populations. Its effects may be complicated by other factors and exacerbated by inbreeding. Examples are given of instances in which disease appears to be playing a part in reducing the numbers of threatened birds or retarding their rate of recovery or spread. There is a need for greater attention to be paid to the role of disease in wild birds, to the provision of more information on this subject and to the establishment of databases and reference collections.

THE IMPACT OF DISEASE ON BIRDS

Many organisms are capable of producing disease in birds. There is much documented information on the pathogens of domestic birds, particularly the fowl (*Gallus domesticus*), and the effect that they have on their host. Useful reference texts in this regard include those by Gordon (1977) and Hofstad *et al.* (1984). Insofar as wild (non-domestic) birds are concerned there is less information available, but nevertheless ample evidence that in captivity pathogens can and do cause disease and death, sometimes of epizootic (epidemic) proportions (Arnall & Keymer 1975; Cooper 1978; Harrison & Harrison 1986; Petrak 1982).

Data on captive birds are of relevance to free-living populations for two reasons:

1. Some species are bred in captivity for subsequent release (see, for example, Carpenter *et al.*, Jones *et al.*, this volume): morbidity or mortality due to disease can seriously hamper such programmes and may even prejudice free-living populations if pathogenic organisms are introduced with the birds at release.
2. If a species proves to be susceptible to an infectious disease when in captivity, it is highly likely that the same organism could prove pathogenic in the wild.

Field biologists should not, therefore, be misled into thinking that information about disease gained from work with birds in captivity—for example, in zoos or private collections—is of no relevance to their studies on free-living populations. It is also easy to forget that a wild bird has an internal ecosystem, consisting of bacteria and other organisms, that is as complex as the external ecosystem in which it lives, and just as sensitive to disruption.

Substantially less information exists on the role of infectious disease in free-living avian populations, even those that are not threatened. This is partly because sick and dead wild birds are often not detected, and partly because in many countries there is no system whereby those birds that are found can be meaningfully examined and the findings recorded. Added to this, few people with a veterinary background or training in avian pathology are attached to units working in the field. Wildlife biologists usually have little specific training in, or experience of, disease and may therefore not suspect or diagnose it. For instance, an owl may be found dead on the road, with multiple injuries, but the presence of a bacterial infection—which may have predisposed to the accident—is only likely to be discovered if the carcass is subjected to a post-mortem examination and supporting laboratory tests. Although there are many reports and descriptions of infectious and parasitic disease in individual wild (free-living) birds it is the outbreaks that affect large populations that attract the greatest attention and interest. There are many examples. Perhaps the most spectacular are those documented by the National Wildlife Health Research Center in the USA: for instance, avian cholera (*Pasteurella* infection) and botulism (*Clostridium botulinum* toxicity) can be responsible for hundreds of thousands of deaths in waterfowl (Friend 1987; Mulcahy *et al.* 1988). Such outbreaks usually occur in gregarious birds, and the examples given are 'population dependent' diseases, the prevalence of which rises as the number of birds in a group increases. Individual wild birds *do* succumb to disease and such cases are of interest and importance, but their impact on populations is usually negligible. This should not be assumed, however. As has been pointed out (V. R. Simpson, pers. comm.), thousands of common birds may die in, for example, a botulism outbreak with no obvious effect on the population(s) but if only two or three Bitterns (*Botaurus stellaris*) were to succumb, the loss to the (British) national population would be substantial.

In some cases infectious or parasitic disease has an effect, but in terms of breeding success rather than mortality. For example, the nematode worm *Trichostrongylus tenuis* can reduce production in the Red Grouse (*Lagopus scoticus*) (Hudson 1986), but such effects are not always easy to detect and evaluate. Recently there has been an upsurge of interest amongst ecologists in pathogenic organisms: Dobson & Hudson (1986) pointed out '. . . parasites and pathogens form important components in the structure of ecological communities . . . they may have serious implications for conservation and management'. They warn, however, that in each of the cases they cite (of disease influencing numbers or fecundity of wildlife) . . . the presence of the pathogen was only confirmed after its effects had been studied in some detail'.

In a later paper May (1988) pursued this theme in more detail and stated 'Given the conspicuous role that diseases have played, and in many parts of the world continue to play, in human demography, it is surprising that ecologists have given so little attention to the way diseases may affect the distribution and abundance of other animals and plants'. After reference to examples, he said, 'In short, infectious diseases are important in the ecology and biogeography of many species, and they are correspondingly important in conservation biology',

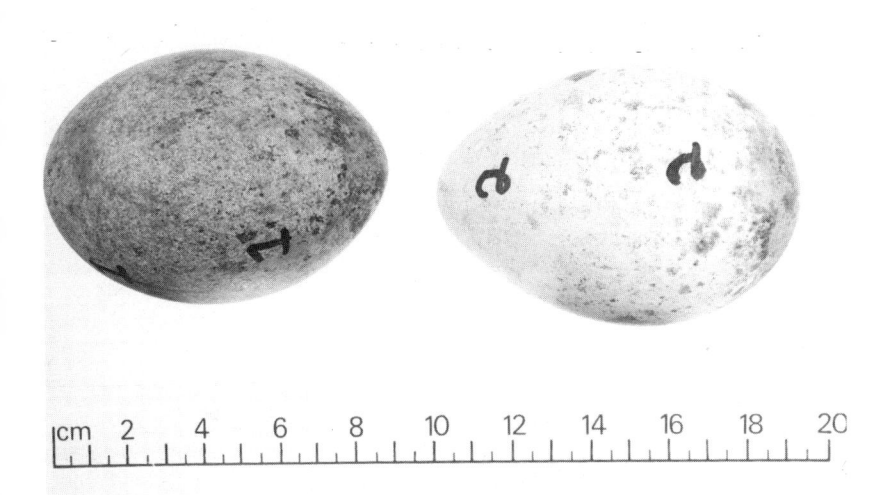

Figure 1: Failure of eggs to hatch may be indicative of infectious disease or contamination. These Black Vulture (*Aegypius monachus*) eggs, collected in Mallorca in 1984, are shown ready for pathological and toxicological analysis. (*Photo*: J. E. Cooper)

but went on to reiterate that this field of research is often not easy and can present many problems. The particular need to monitor infectious disease in wildlife was emphasized by Plowright (1988) who stressed the importance of serological studies as well as surveys and observation of population trends.

It can be particularly difficult to evaluate disease in 'threatened' birds i.e. species that fall into the IUCN (International Union for Conservation of Nature) categories of endangered, vulnerable, indeterminate, rare or insufficiently known (Collar & Stuart 1985). Such populations are, by definition, already under pressure—often because of habitat destruction or toxic chemicals or a combination of other factors. If deaths occur and a disease is diagnosed it may not be possible to say whether this was *per se* responsible for death, one of a number of factors contributing to death, or of no significance at all. The picture that emerges may even depend upon who is investigating the problem: thus, a veterinarian may implicate disease and underestimate the importance of (for example) the bird's poor condition and damaged plumage, while an ecologist might focus on the latter, attributing death to starvation, and ignore (or perhaps be unaware of) the presence of lesions such as abscesses in the bird's lungs or excessive urates in the kidneys. As Ralph & van Riper (1985) stated, 'The importance of bird diseases is one factor in extinctions that most ornithologists feel somewhat uncertain in assessing. This is because many of these diseases could have had their effect many years ago, been brief in their duration, and devastating in their effect. Few investigators have had the fortune to be present during an epidemic, and fewer still have had the tools to monitor the causes and effects'. For this reason it is desirable to have a multidisciplinary approach to morbidity and mortality: a more accurate diagnosis is likely to be achieved if the veterinarian and biologist work together.

THE ROLE OF DISEASE IN EXTINCTION

Despite the recognition for many centuries of diseases affecting birds, it is only in the past few decades that any attention has been paid to their possible role in extinction. Jackson (1977) stated that 'Diseases and parasites are always a threat to any population but are often difficult to detect and identify: they can be disastrous to small isolated populations of endangered species'. It is not easy to obtain data to support the latter statement. Perhaps the earliest suggestion that disease might be involved in the disappearance of a species can be attributed to Brasil (1912) who queried whether it might be a factor in the rapid disappearance of the Réunion Starling (*Fregilupus varius*). Many years later Warner (1968) postulated that the extinction of so many species of Hawaiian birds could be due to introduced diseases such as malaria and avian pox. This theory was pursued in earnest by van Riper and others (see later). In 1971 Rowan, and in 1974 Markus, put forward the hypothesis that arthropod-borne disease was a limiting factor in the distribution of African birds, but provided very little scientific evidence to support this. Temple (1978) discussed the possible influence of infectious and parasitic disease on avian populations and stressed that, in order to cause a decline, this (like any other factor) must cause a reduction in either survivorship or fecundity in the population. Studies on the threatened Mauritius Kestrel (*Falco punctatus*) prompted Cooper et al. (1981) to suggest that this species—and possibly others on Mauritius—might be particularly susceptible to infectious disease and that the situation could be exacerbated by inbreeding (Cooper 1979). The latter was echoed by Temple (1986) who described the recovery of the kestrel 'from an extreme population bottleneck', and drew attention to the species' high inbreeding coefficient and the possible effect that this might have on mortality rates. So-called 'genetic impoverishment' has been postulated as an exacerbating factor in disease in other small populations (May 1988) and is worthy of more attention.

The question of Mascarene species was also addressed by Cheke (1987) who drew attention to the work of Peirce (1979) and Peirce et al. (1977) which revealed that certain blood parasites of birds had been introduced to the Mascarenes. Cheke postulated that avian malaria on Mauritius might be restricted to lower regions, where the vector, *Culex pipiens quinquefasciatus*, also an introduced species, was to be found. Jones & Owadally (1985) drew attention to the various factors that have probably contributed to the decline of the Mauritius Kestrel: they stressed the need to continue to monitor this species for diseases and pathogens and to maintain a veterinary input into their project so that health problems could be dealt with promptly.

Research on the island of Guam by Savidge (1986, 1987) provided 'a rare opportunity to study the decline and impending extinction of an entire forest avifauna'. Investigations carried out included the sampling of domestic, native and introduced birds for micro-organisms, and the use of 'sentinels' in an attempt to detect pathogens in the forest environment. The surveys proved negative— the author's conclusions were that an introduced snake (*Boiga irregularis*) was probably responsible for the decline in the avifauna—but the methods used provide an excellent example of how disease studies should be incorporated into any investigations into the decline of threatened bird populations.

The most detailed studies to date on the role of disease in threatened birds have been by van Riper and his colleagues working in Hawaii. They have produced convincing evidence to confirm the observations of Warner (1968) that extinctions of birds on those islands since the 1920s were due to infections spread by introduced mosquitoes (van Riper *et al.* 1986). This conclusion followed extensive study of the Hawaiian avifauna and its parasites and pathogens (van Riper & van Riper 1985). The results of their work can be summarized as follows. Avian pox and malaria (*Plasmodium* infection) have played a significant part in regulating avian populations on Hawaii. In the case of pox some of the native birds appear to have developed a degree of resistance, but the malaria parasite continues to exercise an important influence, largely by contributing to a restriction of native birds to the higher forest areas where the prevalence of infection is lower.

Many ornithologists and ecologists are now aware of the need to investigate the role of disease in the decline of avian populations in addition to more widely recognized factors such as habitat alteration, pollution, exotic introductions and human exploitation. This approach is not only being applied on islands and elsewhere to species that are threatened with extinction, but also to localized populations that are declining in numbers and to research on threatened species in captivity. Some examples of studies that have addressed this question are given in *Table 1*.

CONCLUSIONS

From the limited information available, some of it based on the studies listed in *Table 1*, it appears that infectious and parasitic diseases can influence wild bird populations either by causing premature death or by reducing reproductive performance. The indications are that disease is likely to have the greatest impact on a naive population i.e. one that has not previously encountered the infection. This was the case in the birds studied by van Riper *et al.* (1986) and there is evidence of the susceptibility to pathogens of some threatened species from other quarters: for example, Snyder *et al.* (1985) reported deaths in captive Pink Pigeons (*Nesoenas* (= *Columba*) *mayeri*) at Albuquerque Zoo (USA) due to a *Herpesvirus* transmitted to them by foster doves (*Columba livia*). The Pink Pigeons, which had come from Mauritius, appear to have had no previous experience of this organism, and it is clear that introduction of the *Herpesvirus* to Mauritius might have had disastrous consequences. Another example concerning columbiform birds was reported by Harmon *et al.* (1987) who found the protozoan parasite *Trichomonas gallinae* only in doves on the Galapagos that were on islands colonized by domestic pigeons. It is assumed that the latter introduced the parasite. The importance of minimizing the risk of introducing potential pathogens, by protecting threatened populations and carrying out regular monitoring (Cooper 1988), is discussed in more detail in subsequent papers.

There is an urgent need for action to minimize the risks of spread of infectious disease from one locality to another. Many species are declining at an alarming rate: a recent estimate suggested that over 1000 of the world's bird species are at risk of extinction (Anon 1988). At the same time, novel pathogens and/or their vectors can be spread with increasing ease, mainly as a result of more frequent air travel. It is worth noting that on Guam the number of species of mosquito increased from 5 to 35 in only 40 years. The spread of avian pathogens is not, of course, of relevance only to wild birds. The spread from one country

Table 1: Examples of studies on wild birds that include disease investigations.

Locality of study	Species of bird	Authors
Indian Ocean		
Mauritius	Mauritius Kestrel (*Falco punctatus*)	Cooper, Jones & Owadally (1981)
	Pink Pigeon (*Nesoenas = Columba mayeri*)	Jones *et al.* (this volume)
Seychelles	Various	Hoogstraal & Feare (1984)
Europe		
West Germany	Peregrine (*Falco peregrinus*)	Schilling *et al.* (1981)
Great Britain	Goshawk (*Accipiter gentilis*)	Cooper & Petty (1988)
	Barn Owl (*Tyto alba*)	Cooper (1987)
	Merlin (*Falco columbarius*)	Cooper & Forbes (1986)
	Manx Shearwater (*Puffinus puffinus*)	Nuttall *et al.* (1982, 1985)
	Red Grouse (*Lagopus lagopus scoticus*)	Wilson & Wilson (1978) Hudson (1986)
	Hawaiian Goose (*Branta sandvicensis*)	Kear (1977)
	Rothschild's Mynah (*Leucopsar rothschildi*)	Kear (1977)
	Chough (*Pyrrhocorax pyrrhocorax*)	Bignal *et al.* (1987)
Jersey	Rodrigues Fody (*Fodia flavicans*) and other species	Cooper and others (unpublished work)
Yugoslavia	Various	Mikuska *et al.* (1986)
Asia		
Thailand	Green Peafowl (*Pavo muticus*)	Hillgarth (this volume)
Papua-New Guinea	Various	Varghese & Yayabu (1981)
Philippines	Philippine Eagle (*Pithecophaga jefferyi*)	Cooper and others (unpublished work)
America		
United States	Whooping Crane (*Grus americana*)	Carpenter *et al.* (this volume)
	Bald Eagle (*Haliaeetus leucocephalus*)	Grubb *et al.* (1986)
	Cliff Swallow (*Hirundo pyrrhonota*)	Emlen (1986)
	Wild Turkey (*Meleagris gallopavo*)	Kutz & Crawford (1987) Davidson *et al.* (1985)
	Goshawk (*Accipiter gentilis*)	Redig *et al.* (1980)
Canada	Various	Hunter (this volume)
Puerto Rico	Pearly-eyed Thrasher (*Margarops fuscatus*)	Arendt (1985) Uhazy and Arendt (1986)
Peru and Galapagos	Blue-footed Booby (*Scula nebouxi*)	Duffy & Duffy (1986)
Falklands	Rockhopper Penguin (*Eudyptes crestatus*)	Keymer (1987)

Table 1—continued.

Locality of study	Species of bird	Authors
America *contd.*		
Guam	Various, including Guam Rail (*Rallus owsta*)	Savidge (1986)
Hawaii	Various, including Hawaiian Crow (*Corvus hawaiiensis*)	Jenkins *et al* (this volume) van Riper & van Riper (1985)
	Hawaiian goose (*Branta sandvicensis*)	Gassman-Duvall (1987)
Africa		
Kenya	Various raptors	Cooper (1973)
South Africa	Jackass Penguin (*Spheniscus demersus*)	Daturi (1986)
Australasia		
Australia	Various	McOrist (this volume)
	Cattle Egret (*Ardeola ibis*)	McKilligan (1987)
New Zealand	Kiwis (*Apteryx* spp.)	Clark (1981)

to another of infectious disease can threaten the poultry industry and, in some instances, may pose dangers to human health (Bourne, this volume). Ralph & van Riper's (1985) statement (in the context of Hawaii) that 'It is vital that no new diseases and parasites or their vectors be introduced to the islands', and Watson's (1984) (in the context of the Seychelles) that '... any evidence of widespread diseases in such small insular populations would give serious cause for concern, and ought to be closely investigated', could usefully be applied to all other areas of the world. It is, perhaps, pertinent to remember that microbes and parasites are no less 'exotic organisms' than are introduced birds, mammals or other species: the concern shown over the indiscriminate movement of these vertebrates (Courtenay & Robins 1975) should be applied to *all* introductions, regardless of size or taxonomic position. This must be borne in mind in addition to humanitarian considerations when, as not infrequently happens, it is suggested that micro-organisms might be used to control introduced species, especially on islands (Dobson 1988).

Clearly much more must be done to foster an awareness of the possible role of disease in wild bird populations. This requires education of all those likely to be involved—avian biologists, field workers, veterinarians and administrators. A useful way of disseminating information is in the form of articles and leaflets. One small step in this direction was the production by ICBP of guidelines for those dealing with threatened birds (Cooper 1983). Furtherance of our knowledge of the subject will come only from research and the collation of data. Insofar as the former is concerned, as was illustrated earlier, some workers are already investigating the role of disease in specific populations, and both zoologists and veterinarians are learning to appreciate the value of collaborative research. Collation of data is important if workers are to have ready access to both published and unpublished material: with this in mind a Reference Collection of Endangered Mascarene Specimens has been established (Cooper & Jones 1986). This consists of carcasses and tissues, eggshells and their contents, paraffin blocks and slides, reprints, photomicrographs and radiographs—all from animals (not only birds) that have died on the Mascarene islands or in one of the captive breeding programmes for these species elsewhere in the world. The main aim of the Collection is to provide a central registry for research on disease and pathology in endangered Mascarene species, but the specimens are also available for such traditional museum studies as morphometrics, osteology and myology. The establishment of similar reference collections elsewhere is clearly desirable, as is the compilation of lists and maps detailing the geographical distribution of diseases in order to assist those involved in field work or the movement of birds from one locality to another.

In addition to the dissemination of information and the collection of material there is an urgent need for more research—a plea that is echoed by many authors in this book and which is reiterated in the Conclusions. Far too little work has been carried out on the role of micro-organisms in wild birds: there is a particular need to monitor threatened populations and to improve methods of so doing. Some pathogens might well be playing a part in reducing the viability or fecundity of certain species but because no attempts have been made to isolate or detect the organisms their role is not appreciated. For example, do avian paramyxoviruses (PMV) affect birds of prey and other species in Britain? PMV1 has spread to pigeons in many parts of the country: might it pose a threat to Peregrines (*Falco peregrinus*) and other predators? Similarly, louping ill virus is known to affect the Red Grouse (*Lagopus lagopus scoticus*) but might it not also infect other ground-nesting moorland species such as the Merlin (*Falco columbarius*) and Dotterel (*Eudromias morinellus*)? If these sorts of questions can be asked in a relatively small country with a well developed network of laboratories and veterinary investigation centres and a large human population with a keen interest in wildlife, especially birds, how many more unsolved problems must there be in those Third World countries in which so many of the rarest species survive? There is clearly a need for more research and when, in another two or three decades, the history of the role of pathogens in threatened avian populations comes to be rewritten, the picture that emerges may be very different.

REFERENCES

ANON 1988. Red data alert: eleven percent of the World's birds threatened. *World Birdwatch* **10** (2), 1–2.

ARENDT, W. J. 1985. *Philornis* ectoparasitism of pearly-eyed thrashers. I. Impact on growth and development of nestlings. *Auk* **102**: 270–80.

ARNALL, L. & KEYMER, I. F. 1975. (eds). *Bird Diseases*. Baillière Tindall, London.

BIGNAL, E., BIGNAL, S. & STILL, E. 1987. Gapeworm infection in choughs. *Ringing and Migration* **8**: 56–8.

BRASIL, L. 1912. Un oiseau éteint de la Réunion, *Fregilupus varius* (Bodd.). *Bull. Soc. Linn. Normandie Sér.* **6**: 16–29.

CHEKE, A. S. 1987. An ecological history of the Mascarene Islands, with particular reference to extinctions and introductions of land vertebrates. *In*: Diamond, A. W. (ed.). *Studies on Mascarene Island Birds*. Cambridge University Press.

CLARK, W. C. 1981. Parasites of Kiwis. *In*: Fowler, M. E. (ed.). *Wildlife Diseases of the Pacific Basin and Other Countries*. Wildlife Disease Association.

COLLAR, N. J. & STUART, S. N. 1985. *Threatened Birds of Africa and Related Islands. The ICBP/IUCN Red Data Book. Part I*. ICBP/IUCN, Cambridge.

COOPER, J. E. 1973. Post-mortem findings in East African birds of prey. *J. Wildl. Dis.* **9**: 368–75.

COOPER, J. E. 1978. *Veterinary Aspects of Captive Birds of Prey*. Standfast Press, Glos.

COOPER, J. E. 1979. An oviduct adenocarcinoma in a Mauritius kestrel (*Falco punctatus*). *Avian Path.* **8**: 187–91.

COOPER, J. E. 1983. *Guideline Procedures for Investigating Mortality in Endangered Birds.* International Council for Bird Preservation, Cambridge.

COOPER, J. E. 1987. Barn owl project—post-mortem findings. *In*: Shawyer, C. R. (ed.). *The Barn Owl in the British Isles.* The Hawk Trust, London.

COOPER, J. E. (1988). Disease transfer and susceptibility in birds. Paper presented at ICBP/WFT Meeting on the Value of Re-Introduction to Bird Conservation. The Wildfowl Trust, Slimbridge, 1988.

COOPER, J. E. & FORBES, N. A. 1986. Studies on morbidity and mortality in the merlin (*Falco columbarius*). *Vet. Rec.* **118**: 232–5.

COOPER, J. E. & JONES, C. G. 1986. A reference collection of endangered Mascarene specimens. *Linnean* **2**: 32–7.

COOPER, J. E., JONES, C. G. & OWADALLY, A. W. 1981. Morbidity and mortality in the Mauritius kestrel (*Falco punctatus*). *In*: Cooper, J. E. & Greenwood A. G. (eds). *Recent Advances in the Study of Raptor Diseases.* Chiron Publications, Keighley.

COOPER, J. E. & PETTY, S. J. 1988. Trichomoniasis in free-living goshawks *Accipiter gentilis gentilis* from Great Britain. *J. Wildl. Dis.* **24**: 80–7.

COURTENAY, W. R. & ROBINS, C. R. 1975. Exotic organisms: an unsolved, complex problem. *Bio Science* **25**: 306–13.

DATURI, A. 1986. A preliminary study of tick populations in Jackass Penguin nests on Marcus Island, South Africa. *Ostrich* **57**: 95–100.

DAVIDSON, W. R., NETTLES, V. F., COUVILLON, C. E. & HOWERTH, E. W. 1985. Diseases diagnosed in wild turkeys (*Meleagris gallopavo*) of the Southeastern United States. *J. Wildl. Dis.* **21**: 386–90.

DOBSON, A. P. 1988. Restoring island ecosystems: the potential of parasites to control introduced mammals. *Conservation Biology* **2**: 31–40.

DOBSON, A. P. & HUDSON, P. J. 1986. Parasites, disease and the structure of ecological communities. *TREE* **1**: 11–14.

DUFFY, D. C. & DUFFY, M. J. C. D. 1986. Tick parasitism at nesting colonies of blue-footed boobies in Peru and Galapagos. *Condor* **88**: 242–244.

EMLEN, J. T. 1986. Responses of breeding cliff swallows to nidicolous parasite infestations. *Condor* **88**: 110–11.

FRIEND, M. 1987. (ed.). *Field Guide to Wildlife Diseases Volume I. General Field Procedures and Diseases of Migrating Birds.* U.S. Department of the Interior, Fish and Wildlife Service, Washington DC.

GASSMAN-DUVALL, L. R. 1987. An acute *Cyathostoma bronchialis* outbreak in the Hawaiian goose and other parasite findings. *Proceedings of 1st International Conference of Zoological and Avian Medicine.* AAV/AAZV, Hawaii, 1987.

GORDON, R. F. 1977. (ed.). *Poultry Diseases.* Baillière Tindall, London.

GRUBB, T. G., EAKLE, W. L. & TUGGLE, B. N. 1986. *Haematosiphon inodorus* (Hemiptera: Cimicidae) in a nest of a bald eagle (*Haliaeetus leucocephalus*) in Arizona. *J. Wildl. Dis.* **22**: 125–7.

HARMON, W. M., CLARK, W. A., HAWBECKER, A. C. & STAFFORD, M. 1987. *Trichomonas gallinae* in columbiform birds from the Galapagos Islands. *J. Wildl. Dis.* **23**: 492–4.

HARRISON, G. J. & HARRISON, L. R. 1986. (eds). *Clinical Avian Medicine and Surgery.* W. B. Saunders, Philadelphia.

HOFSTAD, M. S., BARNES, H. J., CALNEK, B. W., REID, W. M. & YODER, H. W. 1984. (eds). *Diseases of Poultry.* Iowa State University Press, Ames.

HOOGSTRAAL, H. & FEARE, C. J. 1984. Ticks and tick borne viruses. *In*: Stoddard, D. R. (ed.). *Biography and Ecology of the Seychelles Islands.* Dr. W. Junk, The Hague.

HUDSON, P. J. 1986. The effect of a parasitic nematode on the breeding production of red grouse. *J. Anim. Ecol.* **55**: 85–92

JACKSON, J. A. 1977. Alleviating problems of competition, predation, parasitism and disease in endangered birds. A review. *In*: Temple, S. A. (ed.). *Endangered Birds, Management Techniques for Preserving Threatened Species.* University of Wisconsin Press.

JONES, C. G. & OWADALLY, A. W. 1985. The status, ecology and conservation of the

Mauritius kestrel. *In*: Newton, I. & Chancellor, R. D. (eds). *Conservation Studies on Raptors*. ICBP Technical Publication No. 5. ICBP, Cambridge.

KEAR, J. 1977. The problems of breeding endangered species in captivity. *Int. Zoo. Yb.* **17**: 5–14.

KEYMER, I. F. 1987. *An Investigation of Rockhopper Penguin (Eudyptes crestatus) Mortality in the Falklands during the 1985–1986 Breeding Season*. Falkland Islands Foundation Project Report.

KUTZ, R. S. & CRAWFORD, J. A. 1987. Prevalence of poxvirus in a population of Merriam's wild turkeys in Oregon. *J. Wildl. Dis.* **23**: 306–7.

MCKILLIGAN, N. 1987. Causes of nesting loss in the cattle egret *Ardeola ibis* in eastern Australia with special reference to the pathogenicity of the tick *Argas (Persicargas) robertsi* to nestlings. *Aust. J. Ecol.* **12**: 9–16.

MARKUS, M. B. 1974. Arthropod-borne disease as a possible factor limiting the distribution of birds. *Int. J. Parasit.* **4**: 609–12.

MAY, R. M. 1988. Conservation and disease. *Conservation Biology* **2**: 28–36.

MIKUSKA, J., MIKUSKA, T., PELLE, I. & PELLE, Z. 1986. Ugibanje ptica na slanom kopovu kod novog beceja Ijeti 1982. Godine. *Larus* **36–37**, 311–15.

MULCAHY, D., WARPINSKI, P., BENJAMIN, D. & HAMILTON, D. 1988. Avian Cholera and Related Topics: an Annotated Bibliography. *U.S. Fish & Wildlife Service Biol. Rep.* **88**(40).

NUTTALL, P. A., PERRINS, C. M. & HARRAP, K. 1982. Further studies on puffinosis, a disease of the Manx Shearwater (*Puffinus puffinus*). *Can. J. Zool.* **60**: 3462–5.

NUTTALL, P. A., BROOKE, M. DE L. & PERRINS, C. M. 1985. Poxvirus infection of the Manx Shearwater (*Puffinus puffinus*). *J. Wildl. Dis.* **21**: 120–4.

PEIRCE, M. A. 1979. Some additional observations on haematozoa of birds in the Mascarene Islands. *Bull. Brit. Orn. Club* **99**: 68–71.

PEIRCE, M. A., CHEKE, A. S. & CHEKE, R. A. 1977. A survey of blood parasites of birds in the Mascarene Islands, Indian Ocean, with descriptions of two new species and taxonomic discussion. *Ibis* **119**: 451–61.

PETRAK, M. L. 1982. (ed.). *Diseases of Cage and Aviary Birds*. Lea & Febiger, Philadelphia.

PLOWRIGHT, W. 1988. Viruses transmissible between wild and domestic animals. *In*: Smith, G. R. & Hearn, J. P. (eds). *Reproduction and Disease in Captive and Wild Animals*. Symposia of the Zoological Society of London. Number 60. Clarendon Press, Oxford.

RALPH, C. J. & VAN RIPER, C. 1985. Factors affecting Hawaiian birds. *In*: Temple, S. A. (ed.). *Bird Conservation*. University of Wisconsin Press.

REDIG, P. T., FULLER, M. R. & EVANS, D. L. 1980. Prevalence of *Aspergillus fumigatus* in free-living goshawks (*Accipiter gentilis gentilis*). *J. Wild. Dis.* **16**: 169–74.

ROWAN, M. K. 1971. On temperature and disease as limiting factors in distribution. *Ostrich* (Suppl. No. 9): 147–51.

SAVIDGE, J. A. 1986. *The Role of Disease and Predation in the Decline of Guam's Avifauna*. Dissertation, University of Illinois.

SAVIDGE, J. A. 1987. Extinction of an island forest avifauna by an introduced snake. *Ecology* **68**: 660–8.

SCHILLING, F., BÖTTCHER, M. & WALTER, G. 1981. Probleme des Zeckenbefalls bei Nestlingen des Wanderfalken (*Falco peregrinus*). *J. Orn.* **122**: 359–67.

SNYDER, B., THILSTEAD, J., BURGESS, B. & RICHARD, M. 1985. Pigeon Herpesvirus mortalities in foster reared Mauritius pink pigeons. *Abstracts and Papers—1985 Annual Meeting, American Association of Zoo Veterinarians, Arizona*.

TEMPLE, S. A. 1978. (ed.). *Endangered Birds. Management Techniques for Preserving Threatened Species*. University of Wisconsin Press.

TEMPLE, S. A. 1986. Recovery of the endangered Mauritius kestrel from an extreme population bottleneck. *Auk* **103**: 632–3.

UHAZY, L. S. & ARENDT, W. J. 1986. Pathogenesis associated with philornid myiasis (Diptera: Muscidae) on nestling pearly-eyed thrashers (Aves: Mimidae) in the Luquillo Rain Forest, Puerto Rico. *J. Wildl. Dis.* **22**: 224–37.

VAN RIPER, S. G. & VAN RIPER, C. 1985. A summary of known parasites and diseases from the avifauna of the Hawaiian Islands. *In*: Stone, C. P. & Scott, J. M. (eds). *Hawaii's Terrestrial Ecosystems, Preservation and Management*. Co-operative National Park Resources Studies Unit, University of Hawaii.

VAN RIPER, C., VAN RIPER, S. G., GOFF, M. L. & LAIRD, M. 1986. The epizootiology and ecological significance of malaria in Hawaiian land birds. *Ecological Monographs* **56**: 327–44.

VARGHESE, T. & YAYABU, R. 1981. A survey of coccidian and helminth parasites of birds in Papua New Guinea with special reference to the Birds of Paradise. *In*: Fowler, M. E. (ed.). *Wildlife Diseases of the Pacific Basin and other Countries*. Wildlife Disease Association.

WARNER, R. E. 1968. The role of introduced diseases in the extinction of the endemic Hawaiian avifauna. *Condor* **70**: 101–20.

WATSON, J. 1984. Land birds: endangered species on the granite Seychelles. *In*: Stoddart, D. R. (ed.). *Biography and Ecology of the Seychelles Islands*. Dr. W. Junk, The Hague.

WILSON, G. R. & WILSON, L. P. 1978. Haematology, weight and condition of captive red grouse (*Lagopus lagopus scoticus*) infected with caecal threadworm (*Trichostrongylus tenuis*). *Res. vet. Sci.* **25**: 331–6.

FURTHER READING

BEGON, M., HARPER, J. L. & TOWNSEND, C. R. 1986. *Ecology: Individuals, Populations and Communities*. Sinauer, Sunderland. Mass.

BERGER, A. J. 1972. *Hawaiian Birdlife*. The University Press of Hawaii, Honolulu.

COOPER, J. E. 1979. Veterinary care of wild birds. *Anim. Reg. Studies* **2**: 21–9.

DIAMOND, J. & CASE, T. J. 1985. (eds). *Community Ecology*. Harper & Row.

EBENHARD, T. 1988. Introduced birds and mammals and their ecological effects. *Swedish Wildlife Research* **13**: 5–107.

HALLIDAY, T. 1978. *Vanishing Birds: Their Natural History and Conservation*. Sidgwick & Jackson, London.

SCOTT, J. M., KEPLER, C. B., VAN RIPER, C. & FEFER, S. I. 1988. Conservation of Hawaii's vanishing avifauna. *Bio Science* **38**: 238–53.

SIMON, N. & GÉROUDET, P. 1970. *Last Survivors: The Natural History of Animals in Danger of Extinction*. Patrick Stephens, London.

THORNE, E. T. & WILLIAMS, E. S. 1988. Disease and endangered species: the black-footed ferret as a recent example. *Conservation Biology* **2**: 66–74.

SOME DISEASES OF FREE-LIVING AUSTRALIAN BIRDS

STEVEN MCORIST

Veterinary Research Institute, Park Drive, Parkville, Victoria 3052, Australia.

ABSTRACT

Diseases diagnosed during a five-year period in free-living Tawny Frogmouths (*Podargus strigoides*), Nankeen Night Herons (*Nycticorax caledonicus*), Sulphur-crested Cockatoos (*Cacatua galerita*) and Crimson Rosellas (*Platycercus elegans*) in Victoria, Australia, are reviewed.

Arteriosclerosis, traumatic cataracts, nephrosis secondary to traumatic fractures, and post-weaning starvation were diagnosed in Tawny Frogmouths. Nankeen Night Herons suffered parasitic proventriculitis caused by a *Contracaecum* sp., peritonitis and starvation. Sulphur-crested Cockatoos in one flock exhibited more than 80 percent mortality in a one-year period: affected birds showed gross and histological lesions of psittacine beak and feather dystrophy, a virus-associated disease. Birds from a flock of Crimson Rosellas also had lesions of this disease. Psittacine beak and feather dystrophy thus represents a significant disease threat to threatened populations of Australian psittacine birds. Another flock of Crimson Rosellas suffered approximately 50 percent mortality over a two-year period. Birds from this flock had histological lesions of hepatitis and nephritis, possibly due to a plant or mould toxin.

INTRODUCTION

Nineteen Orders of native bird occur in Australia, with particular diversity among psittacines and passerines. Research on wild birds by groups in universities, government departments and elsewhere has concentrated on ecological aspects. No reference or management centre for threatened bird populations has yet emerged, although some recent research has extended into this area. Recent studies have been made into the ecology of threatened populations of the Gouldian Finch (*Chloebia gouldiae*), Ground Parrot (*Pezoporus wallicus*), Orange-bellied Parrot (*Neophema chrysogaster*), and Little Penguin (*Eudyptula minor*). Only in the last-mentioned study has the role of disease been examined.

As part of a more general survey of the diseases of free-living birds in Victoria, the following birds were studied: Tawny Frogmouth (*Podargus strigoides*: Caprimulgiformes), Nankeen Night Heron (*Nycticorax caledonicus*: Ardeiformes), Sulphur-crested Cockatoo (*Cacatua galerita*: Psittaciformes) and Crimson Rosella (*Platycercus elegans*: Psittaciformes).

Tawny Frogmouths are large nocturnal birds with a diet of large insects and small mammals. Their population dynamics are unknown.

Nankeen Night Herons are nocturnal river feeders which, in common with many other Australian waterbirds, can vary greatly in population density. Exuberant breeding can occur in response to seasonal flooding (Marshall et al 1982); however, the nature of subsequent population declines is not known.

Cockatoos and rosellas form nomadic, monospecific flocks throughout Australia. Neither Sulphur-crested Cockatoos nor Crimson Rosellas are threatened; however, several closely related species, such as *Platycercus flavedus* and *Cacatua sanguinea*, have suffered significantly from habitat destruction and illicit trappings.

MATERIALS AND METHODS

Dead or moribund wild birds were collected by local conservation officers for autopsy during 1980–85. Each bird was subjected to a full gross examination. Parasites were identified by staff of the Australian Helminthological Collection, Adelaide, South Australia. Portions of organs were collected into buffered formalin, and 5 μm sections cut and stained by haematoxylin and eosin for histopathological examination. In those birds with feather and skin problems, care was taken to include longitudinal sections of the base of several feathers. In most cases, portions of fresh liver were cultured on blood agar and MacConkey agar for routine bacteriological examination (Scullion, this volume).

Determination of pesticide concentrations in the stomach contents of selected birds was performed by officers of the State Chemistry Laboratory, Melbourne, Victoria. Age was estimated from gonad size.

Eight Tawny Frogmouths were collected in open woodland, three Nankeen Night Herons from riverbanks, and five Sulphur-crested Cockatoos and ten Crimson Rosellas from semi-arable farmland. No assessment of population size was available for the frogmouths or herons. However, a weekly count of one cockatoo flock and two rosella flocks was available for part of the study period. Birds were counted that congregated near grain feed sources.

RESULTS

The findings are summarized in *Table 1*.

Tawny Frogmouths. Gross lesions consisted of bilateral lens opacity in an adult, traumatic fracture of the radius in a second adult, depletion of fat reserves in two juveniles, and serous clots in the pericardial sacs of two further adults.

Histology confirmed traumatic cataracts, with necrosis and vacuolation of both lenses, and corneal ulceration of one eye in the first bird. The second bird had marked necrosis of the proximal tubules of both kidneys, consistent with acute nephrosis, as well as the bone fracture.

Cardiovascular lesions were present in the two birds with pericardial clots, and two others. Marked proliferation of myocytes and fibroblasts within the tunica media of the coronary arteries was a consistent feature. The cephalic arteries of one bird were also affected. Adventitial oedema and lymphocyte infiltration were seen around coronary arteries of two of these birds. Arteriosclerosis was considered the major lesion in these four birds.

The juvenile birds had no obvious disease and were thought to have starved following weaning. No parasites or other diseases were found.

Table 1: Summary of conditions in selected species of Australian birds.

Bird	Findings	Probable cause
Crimson Rosella (*Platycercus elegans*)	Psittacine beak and feather dystrophy	Virus
	Hepatic degeneration	Mycotoxicosis
	Trauma	Caught in mist net
Nankeen Night Heron (*Nycticorax caledonicus*)	Starvation, Gastric parasitism	Seasonal disturbance in food supply
Tawny Frogmouth (*Podargus strigoides*)	Arteriosclerosis	Haemodynamic stress
Boobook Owl (*Ninox novaeseelandiae*)	Arteriosclerosis	Haemodynamic stress

Nankeen Night Herons. Gross lesions consisted of 10 to 20 ascarid nematodes in the proventriculus of two birds, and fibrinous haemorrhages over the intestinal serosa of a third bird. All birds were in poor body condition, with empty stomachs. Histological examination showed that the ascarids were within the mucosa of the proventriculus of the first two birds, with a local inflammatory reaction. These ascarids were identified as *Contracaecum spiculigerum*. Inflammatory peritonitis, probably secondary to intestinal rupture, was evident in the remaining bird; no parasites were found in these lesions. All birds had apparently died of starvation.

Sulphur-crested Cockatoos. The cockatoo flock declined from about 120 to about 20 birds over a nine-month period. More than 40 dead or dying birds were found, nearly all affected by severe feather loss. Gross lesions in the five juveniles autopsied were constriction, stunting or loss of feathers over the body and wings, with beak overgrowth in two. Affected feathers showed epidermal necrosis and basophilic granules within macrophages in the epidermis and pulp, consistent with psittacine beak and feather dystrophy. No other lesions were noted other than poor body condition.

Crimson Rosellas. One flock declined from about 20 birds to 10 birds over a 20-month period. Gross and histological lesions in the four birds autopsied from this flock were similar to those described above for psittacine beak and feather dystrophy. Affected rosellas were usually found alive, but weak and unable to fly due to feather loss.

Another flock showed a reduction in numbers from about 30 to 15 over a 24-month period. Several birds were found dying, but no gross lesions were seen in the five autopsied. Histological examination showed moderate to severe hepatocyte necrosis, fibrosis and lymphocytic foci within all the livers, and tubular necrosis and cast formation in the kidneys of three birds. The cause of this hepatitis/nephritis syndrome was not determined, but a plant or mould toxicity was suspected. No pesticides were detected in these or other birds.

A further Crimson Rosella with gross haemorrhages and traumatic fractures was received, following its capture in a mist net.

DISCUSSION

Birds belonging to three Orders were studied; therefore different disease patterns

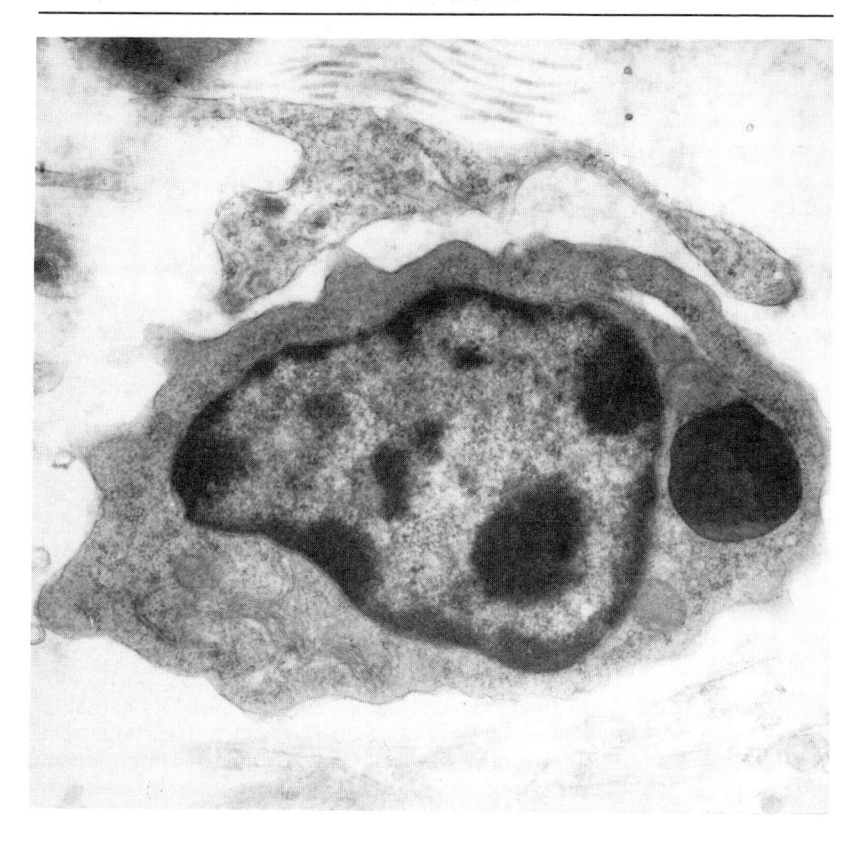

Figure 1: Psittacine beak and feather dystrophy. Section of a feather from a wild-caught Sulphur-crested Cockatoo (*Cacatua galerita*). The cell is a macrophage containing an intracytoplasmic inclusion body (= virus particles). (*Photo:* McOrist)

are evident. Frogmouths showed conditions similar to those described for raptors, the herons died of starvation, and cockatoos and rosellas has infectious and toxic diseases.

Arterial lesions are common in owls and falcons (Cooper & Pomerance 1982). Their occurrence in frogmouths suggests that damaging haemodynamic stresses on arteries may be common to all birds. Arteriosclerosis can progress rapidly in birds, due to the large fibroblast population within the tunica media of their arteries (Cheville 1983). Ocular lesions and nephrosis associated with stressful trauma are also common in raptors (Murphy *et al.* 1982). Viral hepatitis has been reported in a frogmouth (Reece *et al.* 1985).

The herons examined had lesions consistent with reduced food availability. *Contracaecum* spp. are common parasites of Australian waterbirds (Johnston & Mawson 1941); however, their direct pathogenic effect is probably low (Greve *et al.* 1986). Fluctuations in waterbird populations are probably part of a natural ecosystem; however, they are also associated with changes in the occurrence of human arborvirus infections, of which many waterbirds are carriers (Marshall

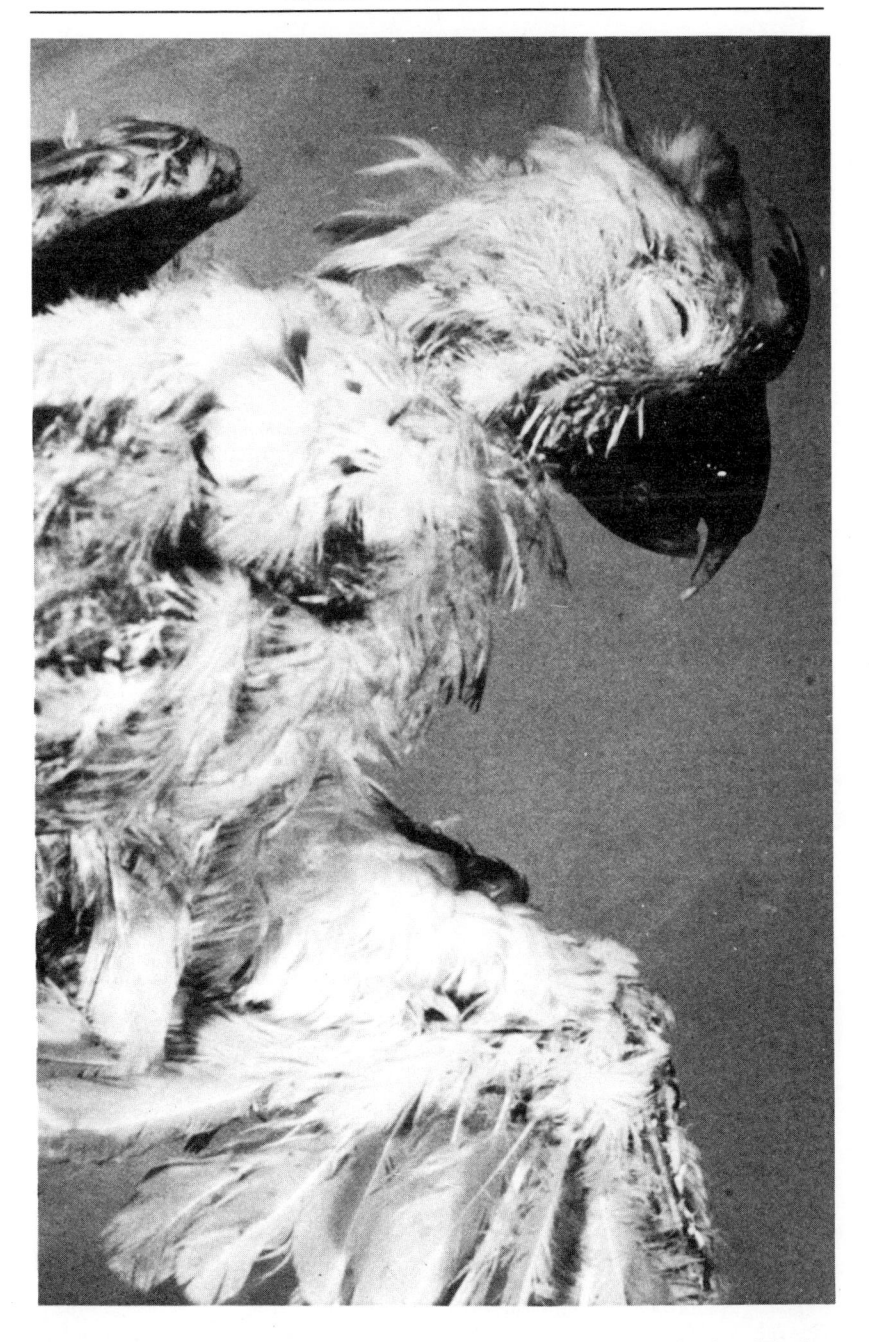

Figure 2: Displaced, broken and abnormal feathers due to psittacine beak and feather dystrophy, shown here in a free-living Sulphur-crested Cockatoo (*Cacatua galerita*). (*Photo*: McOrist)

et al. 1982). Close monitoring of the disease status of these birds is therefore warranted.

Psittacine beak and feather dystrophy (PBFD) is a virus-associated disease, previously described as affecting only 10 to 20 percent of wild Sulphur-crested Cockatoos in certain flocks (McOrist *et al.* 1984). It is assumed that many of the apparent reductions in flock sizes in this study were due to mortality and morbidity rather than migration and redistribution of birds into other flocks. The findings indicate that the disease is capable of causing severe mortality in avian populations, and of affecting species other than Sulphur-crested Cockatoos. Whilst previous studies of captive birds in Australia (Pass & Perry 1984), the USA (Jacobson *et al.* 1986) and Britain (Cooper *et al.* 1987) had similar findings, this investigation suggests that many threatened populations of free-living psittacines in Australia are at risk from the disease. Some of these birds are also threatened by illicit trapping operations and habitat destruction (Weaver 1982).

To complement the necessary work of ecological studies, it is vital that adequate monitoring of the diseases of wild birds is performed, particularly those in populations under threat. Nationally recognized facilities based on a pathology group with toxicological, microbiological and parasitological disciplines, would form the basis for a wildlife health resource. This could readily link with an active management programme for threatened species. Conservation of the variety of Australian wild birds would be greatly enhanced by such co-operation.

REFERENCES

CHEVILLE, N. F. 1983. *Cell Pathology*. Iowa State University Press, Ames.

COOPER, J. E., GSCHMEISSNER, S., PARSONS, A. J. & COLES B. H. 1987. Psittacine beak and feather disease. *Vet. Rec.* **120**: 287.

COOPER J. E. & POMERANCE, A. 1982. Cardiac lesions in birds of prey. *J. Comp. Path.* **92**: 161–8.

GREVE, J. H., ALBERS, H. F., SUTO, B. & GRIMES, J. 1986. Pathology of gastrointestinal helminthiasis in the brown pelican (*Pelecanus occidentalis*). *Avian Dis.* **30**: 428–87.

JACOBSON, E. R., CLUBB, S., SIMPSON, C., WALSH, M., LOTHROP, C. D., GASKIN, J., BAUER, J., HINES, S., KOLLIAS, G. V., POWLES, P. & HARRISON, G. 1986. Feather and beak dystrophy and necrosis in cockatoos: clinicopathologic evaluations. *J. Am. vet. med. Ass.* **189**: 999–1005.

JOHNSTON, T. H. & MAWSON, P. M. 1941. Ascarid nematodes from Australian birds. *Trans. R. Soc. S. Aust.* **65**: 110–15.

MARSHALL, I. D., BROWN, B. K., KEITH, K., GARD, G. P. & THIBOS, E. 1982. Variation in arbovirus infection rates in species of birds sampled in a serological survey during an encephalitis epidemic in the Murray Valley of south-eastern Australia, February 1974. *Aust. J. Exp. Biol. Med. Sci.* **60**: 471–8.

MCORIST, S., BLACK, D. G., PASS, D. A., SCOTT, P. C. & MARSHALL, J. 1984. Beak and feather dystrophy in wild sulphur-crested cockatoos (*Cacatua galerita*). *J. Wildl. Dis.* **20**: 120–4.

MURPHY, C. J., KERN, I. J., MCKEEVER, K., MCKEEVER, L. & MACCOY, D. 1982. Ocular lesions in free-living raptors. *J. Am. vet. med. Ass.* **181**: 1302–4.

PASS, D. A. & PERRY, R. A. 1984. The pathology of psittacine beak and feather disease. *Aust. Vet. J.* **61**: 69–74.

REECE, R. L., PASS, D. A. & BUTLER, R. 1985. Inclusion body hepatitis in a tawny frogmouth (*Podargus stringoides*: Caprimulgiformes). *Aust. Vet. J.* **62**: 426.

WEAVER, C. M. 1982. Breeding habitats and status of the golden-shouldered parrot *Psephotus chrysopterygius*, in Queensland. *Emu* **82**: 2–6.

THE SIGNIFICANCE OF AVIAN HAEMATOZOA IN CONSERVATION STRATEGIES

M. A. PEIRCE

Corresponding Associate, International Reference Centre for Avian Haematozoa, 16 Westmorland Close, Woosehill, Wokingham, Berkshire RG11 9AZ, England.

ABSTRACT

A brief description is given of the life-cycles and pathogenicity of the more common avian haematozoa. These are discussed in relation to potential disease threats to endangered species, especially on islands, due to ecological factors or introductions of infected alien species. Preventive measures and disease monitoring are proposed in relation to captive breeding and conservation programmes.

INTRODUCTION

Blood parasites have been found in many thousands of birds from around the world covering a wide spectrum of species (Bennett *et al.* 1982). Studies range from the examination of individual birds from the wild or in zoological collections, to surveys in specific areas or the study of a number of birds of a single genus or species. The occurrence of haematozoa is usually restricted by geographic and climatic conditions limiting the distribution of vectors. The degree to which parasites are pathogenic is frequently difficult to assess accurately since sick or dying birds in the wild rapidly fall victim to predators or their carcasses go undetected. Concomitant infections with other disease agents, and ecological factors, may also play significant roles. With an ever-increasing number of birds being threatened with extinction, some populations of which are only just viable, it is important that an understanding of the disease potential of haematozoa is taken into account in formulating conservation strategies.

PARASITE GENERA

Parasites belonging to the genera *Plasmodium*, *Haemoproteus*, *Leucocytozoon* and *Trypanosoma* are the most frequently encountered species. Of these, haemoproteids are the most common since the principal vectors are hippoboscids (Diptera) which maintain a closer host-parasite relationship than most other ornithophilic species. Generally, species of *Haemoproteus* and the sub-genus *Parahaemoproteus* (transmitted by *Culicoides* spp.) are family-specific and often host-specific parasites in their avian hosts. Parasitaemia in peripheral blood is frequently high, and endogenous development (schizogony) may occur in many tissues, although the liver and lungs are the usual predilection sites. Only gametocytes are found in peripheral blood.

Species of *Plasmodium* are transmitted by ornithophilic mosquitoes and have a life-cycle similar to that of *Haemoproteus* in their avian host, but they differ in two basic aspects; endogenous development (exo-erythrocytic schizogony) occurs in a wider range of tissues, and the parasite has an asexual cycle resulting in the presence of schizonts in circulating erythrocytes. When erythrocytic schizonts are present they are a useful indicator in establishing a differential diagnosis since the gametocytes of some *Plasmodium* species are similar to those of haemoproteids.

Leucocytozoids are transmitted primarily by simuliids (Diptera) and thus are absent from coral islands and geographic areas devoid of fast-flowing freshwater streams which are the breeding grounds of the principal vectors. The gametocytes of *Leucocytozoon* spp. may invade either leucocytes or erythrocytes in which, by the time they are mature, the host cell has become greatly hypertrophied. Endogenous development occurs in many tissues.

Trypanosomes occur in a wide spectrum of avian species, and most often as subclinical infections undetectable by simple blood film examination. They are transmitted by a more varied range of vectors than most other haematozoa, which includes hippoboscids, simuliids, *Culicoides*, mosquitoes and mites. The high degree of pleomorphism exhibited by many *Trypanosoma* spp., together with low parasitaemias, frequently make a differential diagnosis difficult. Although little is known regarding the biology of trypanosomes in their avian hosts, most are thought to multiply by binary fission in bone marrow and other sites, as such phenomena are rarely seen in peripheral blood.

Parasites belonging to the genera *Atoxoplasma*, *Lankesterella*, *Hepatozoon* and *Babesia*, although occurring in birds, are not considered to pose any significant clinical or pathological manifestations.

EVIDENCE OF PATHOGENICITY

Field evidence of clinical manifestation caused by haematozoa in free-living avian populations is difficult to acquire. The majority of haematozoan parasites are probably benign in their natural host, although relapses with increased parasitaemia may occur, triggered by hormonal activity during breeding, migration or stress (Haberkorn 1968; Peirce & Mead 1984; Peirce 1981). It is probably only where such conditions occur as concomitant infections with other disease agents that the parasites cause any significant or pathogenic effects on the host. There is little evidence that haematozoa exhibit any degree of immunity between different genera, or species of the same genera. Birds are often infected with two or more species of *Haemoproteus*, *Plasmodium* or *Leucocytozoon*, and infections with at least six different parasites in a single host are not uncommon. Molyneux & Gordon (1975) were able to infect birds experimentally with three different *Trypanosoma* species, and whilst natural infections in birds may occasionally show high parasitaemias there is no evidence of pathogenicity. Observations on retrapped birds in Zambia showed that haematozoan infections persisted for long periods with no evidence of immunity to infection with different parasites (Peirce 1984b).

Some parasites may be pathogenic only in domestic birds. *Plasmodium gallinaceum*, a parasite of Galliformes in Asia, is pathogenic in Domestic Chickens (*Gallus domesticus*) but is not known to be in free-living Junglefowl (*Gallus gallus*) which are the natural hosts. A similar situation occurs with *Leucocytozoon* (*Akiba*) *caulleryi* in the same region.

Of all the *Plasmodium* spp. occurring in birds, by far the most common in terms of the numbers of species susceptible, and global distribution, is *P. relictum* which is considered to be the most pathogenic of all the avian species (Garnham 1966). *P. relictum* is particularly pathogenic in several species of penguins in zoos and also occurs in the wild (Bennett *et al.* 1982). It has also been claimed as instrumental in the demise of Hawaiian birds, particularly Drepaniidae, following its introduction (Warner 1968), although it is possible that concomitant avian pox was equally responsible (Jenkins *et al.*, this volume).

Haemoproteids are not generally considered to be pathogenic despite their frequently high parasitaemias, although Markus & Oosthuizen (1972) reported *H. columbae* to be pathogenic in Pigeons (*Columba livia*) in South Africa.

Leucocytozoon marchouxi was found in a clinically sick Emerald-spotted Wood Dove (*Turtur chalcospilos*) in Zambia (Peirce 1984a), and Garnham (1950) attributed deaths in weaverbird nestlings in Kenya to *Leucocytozoon* infection. Conversely, a study of raptors in Scotland revealed that in Sparrowhawk (*Accipiter nisus*) and Buzzard (*Buteo buteo*) chicks, enormously high parasitaemias with *L. toddi* occurred without any recorded mortality (Peirce 1981; Peirce & Marquiss 1983). Some *Leucocytozoon* species, however, may attack both wild and domestic birds with equal virulence, particularly *L. smithi* (turkeys) and *L. simondi* (ducks and geese). Sometimes a parasite may infect an unnatural host and cause fatal disease, as reported in parakeets in England due to an aberrant *Leucocytozoon* infection (Peirce & Bevan 1977).

HAEMATOZOA IN THREATENED BIRD POPULATIONS

In small relict populations of endangered species, benign host-specific haematozoa may have become extinct due to lack of host access. At the same time these birds will most likely be suffering some degree of stress due to factors such as reduced mate choice, diminished food resources, and habitat loss—particularly in highly territorial species. Under these conditions, infection with less host-specific parasites whether normally benign or not, will probably reach intensities likely to cause fatalities, particularly as other arthropod-borne diseases may be present too.

Island populations may, if maintained in isolation, survive any serious effects from indigenous haematozoa due to limited vector populations, as discussed earlier. On larger and more densely populated islands various factors may effect a change in circumstances. On Mauritius, comparative surveys of avian haematozoa separated by some 60 years indicate that *Haemoproteus* has been largely replaced by *Plasmodium*, although this may be due to mis-diagnosis in the earlier survey (Peirce *et al.* 1977). These apparent changes may be due to the human malaria eradication programme which also might have influenced ornithophilic vector populations, and from introductions of infected birds. So far no evidence has been found of haematozoa in the Mauritius Kestrel (*Falco*

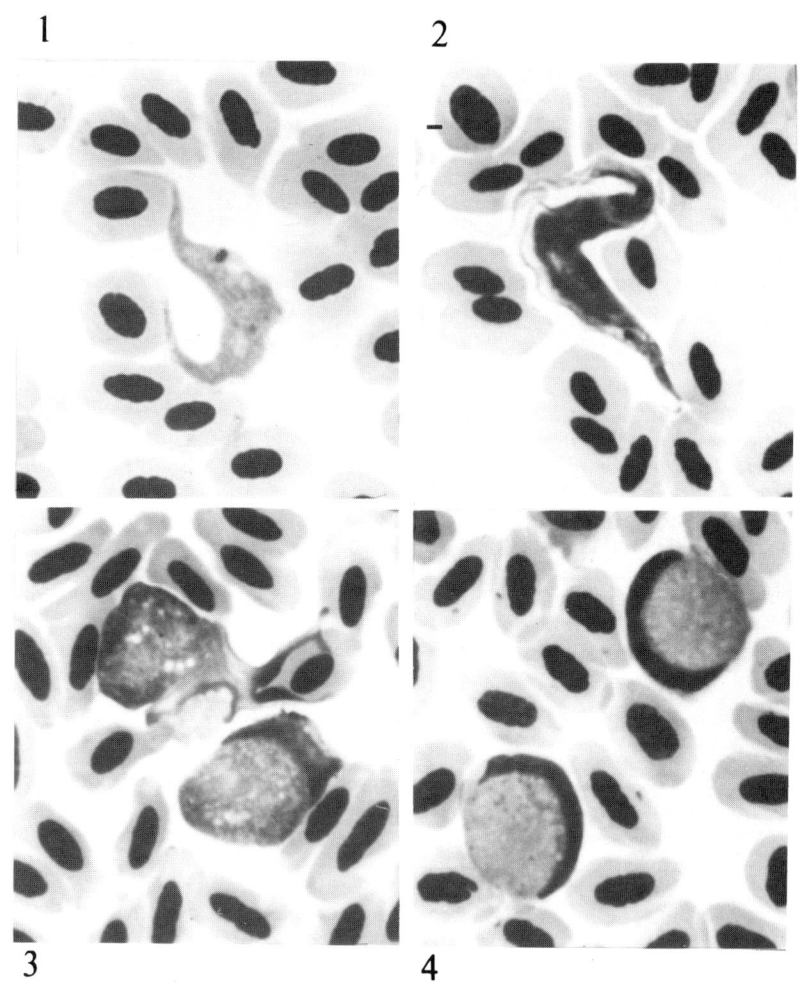

Figure 1: Trypanosoma bouffardi from Blue Waxbill (*Uraeginthus angolensis*).
Figure 2: Trypanosoma pycnonoti from Black-eyed Bulbul (*Pycnonotus barbatus naumanni*).
Figure 3: Leucocytozoon marchouxi from Emerald-spotted Wood Dove (*Turtur chalcospilos*).
Figure 4: Leucocytozoon majoris from Cabanis's Yellow Bunting (*Emberiza cabanisi*).
(*Photos*: Peirce)

Significance of Avian Haematozoa 73

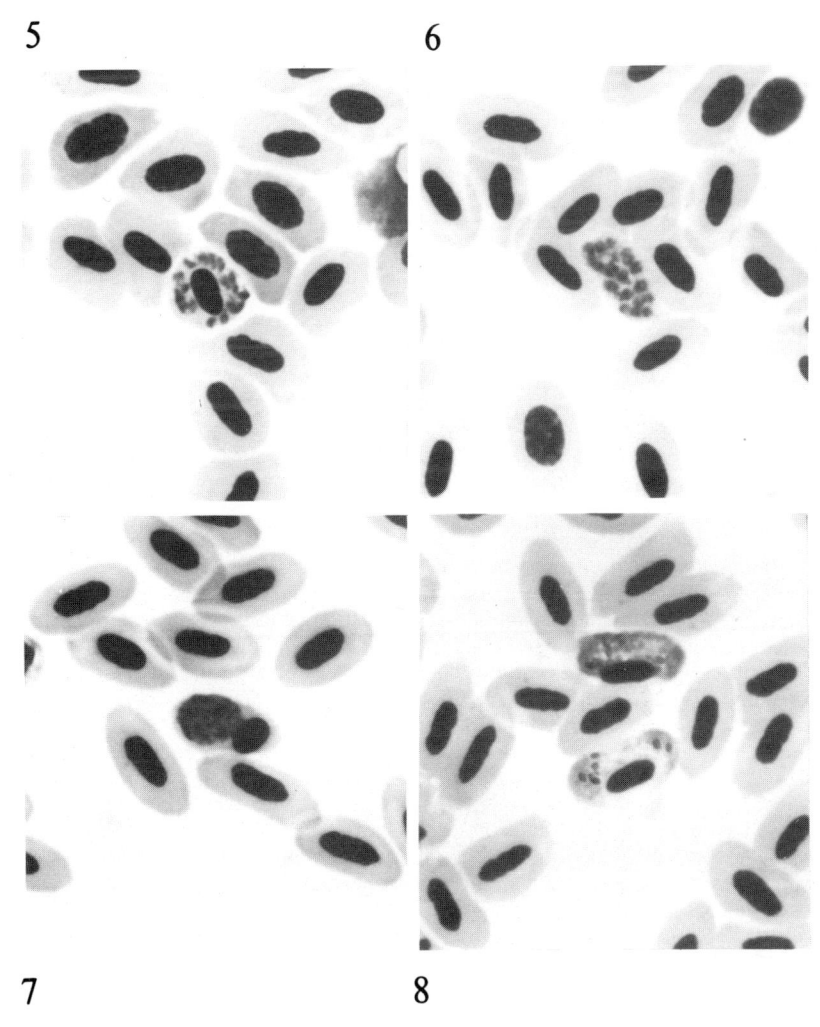

Figure 5: Schizont of *Plasmodium circumflexum* from Blue Waxbill (*Uraeginthus angolensis*).
Figure 6: Schizont of *Plasmodium relictum* in an enucleated erythrocyte from Miombo Grey Tit (*Parus griseiventris*).
Figure 7: Macrogametocyte of *P. relictum* from Miombo Grey Tit (*P. griseiventris*).
Figure 8: Macrogametocyte (upper) and microgametocyte of *Haemoproteus sequeirae* from Scarlet-chested Sunbird (*Nectarinia senegalensis*). (*Photos*: Peirce)

punctatus), but what is thought to be *L. marchouxi* has been observed in the Pink Pigeon (*Nesoenas mayeri*), also on Mauritius (Peirce & Cooper, unpubl. data cited in Cooper *et al.* 1987). *Leucocytozoon* and *Plasmodium* occur in other endemic species in the Mascarenes (Peirce *et al.* 1977; Peirce 1979), some of which are also endangered.

PREVENTIVE MEASURES IN CONSERVATION PROGRAMMES

Many threatened bird species occur in areas where they are not exposed to haematozoan infection due to geographic factors limiting the presence of vectors, such as montane species and those on coral islands. When such birds are removed from their natural environment to captive breeding centres they are then most likely to be exposed to infection with haematozoa and other disease agents. This occurred in drepaniids in Hawaii (Warner 1968; Markus 1974) and is likely to be occurring now in similar situations.

It is difficult to protect captive birds from exposure to disease-transmitting vectors unless they are maintained in fly-proofed aviaries. For the most part this is expensive, impracticable and irrelevant since, if the intention is to return the species to the wild, then it is probably better to limit rather than preclude exposure to vectors and possible infection. Larger birds can be treated with topical applications of insecticide to control ectoparasites, but where such measures are practised, it is most important that a safe product is used, i.e. synthetic pyrethroids. Under no circumstances should toxic agents such as DDT be used, as appears to be the situation currently occurring in some captive breeding centres in Thailand (Hillgarth *et al.*, this volume).

In situations where domestic birds may be kept by local people near captive breeding centres—for example, chickens infected with *P. gallinaceum* in proximity to breeding centres for Galliformes in Asia—care should be taken to restrict or eliminate these birds since they may be host to more virulent strains of the parasite than occur naturally in wild populations. Captive birds infected with a more virulent strain, if released back into the wild, could potentially cause more havoc than would any ecological factors influenced by man.

When foster birds are introduced in captive breeding programmes, particularly when they do not occur indigenously, it is important to ensure that they are first screened for the presence of haematozoa and other likely pathogens (Hunter *et al.*, this volume; Appendix 2).

MONITORING FOR DISEASE

Any wild birds removed from their natural habitat will be under varying degrees of stress, and as little handling as possible is therefore essential. When handling is necessary, samples should be taken for screening. The removal of a small drop of blood from a wing vein or clipped toe can be performed with little or no distress to the bird. Birds bred in captivity should also be monitored for the presence of haematozoa since this will give some indication of the potential risk to which they are being exposed. In rare situations where an infection is deemed to be potentially serious, chemotherapy can be given, but this should be considered only as a last resort.

Today, when there is an ever-increasing demand from the pet trade for exotic bird species, recipient countries should be aware of the potential disease hazards that such importations pose (Laird & Hoogstraal 1975; Ashton & Cooper, Bourne, this volume).

CONCLUSIONS

In their natural environment, wild birds probably do not fall victim to virulent strains of most haematozoan parasites. Concomitant infections with other disease agents may often alter the effect of otherwise benign parasites and in combination become pathogenic. There is always a risk of new disease hazards from imported birds and the accidental introduction of new vectors. Where endangered species are removed from the wild for captive breeding programmes they are more likely to be at risk from infection. Therefore, in conservation and captive breeding programmes due consideration must be given to these factors, and the formulation of strategies must include regular monitoring. The International Reference Centre for Avian Haematozoa is always willing to screen blood smears for the presence of parasites and to co-operate in any study programme.

REFERENCES

BENNETT, G. F., WHITEWAY, M. & WOODWORTH-LYNAS, C. 1982. A host-parasite catalogue of the avian haematozoa. *Memorial Univ. Nfld. Occas. Pap. Biol. No 5*.

COOPER, J. E., NEEDHAM, J. R., APPLEBEE, K. & JONES, C. G. 1987. Clinical and pathological studies on the Mauritian Pink Pigeon *Columba mayeri*. *Ibis* **130**: 57–64.

GARNHAM, P. C. C. 1950. Blood parasites of East African vertebrates, with a brief description of exo-erythrocytic schizogony in *Plasmodium pitmani*. *Parasitology* **40**: 328–37.

GARNHAM, P. C. C. 1966. *Malaria Parasites and Other Haemosporidia*. Blackwell Scientific Publications, Oxford.

HABERKORN, A. 1968. Zur hormonellen Beeinflussung von *Haemoproteus*-Infektionen. *Z. ParasitKde.* **31**: 108–12.

LAIRD, M. & HOOGSTRAAL, H. 1975. Disease hazards associated with bird importations. *Environ. Conserv.* **2**: 119–20.

MARKUS, M. B. 1974. Arthropod-borne disease as a possible factor limiting the distribution of birds. *Int. J. Parasit.* **4**: 609–12.

MARKUS, M. B. & OOSTHUIZEN, J. H. 1972. Pathogenicity of *Haemoproteus columbae*. *Trans. R. Soc. trop. Med. Hyg.* **66**: 186–7.

MOLYNEUX, D. H. & GORDON, E. 1975. Studies on immunity with three species of avian trypanosomes. *Parasitology* **70**: 181–7.

PEIRCE, M. A. 1979. Some additional observations on the haematozoa of birds in the Mascarene Islands. *Bull. Brit. Orn. Cl.* **99**: 68–71.

PEIRCE, M. A. 1981. Current knowledge of the haematozoa of raptors. *In:* Cooper, J. E. & Greenwood, A. G. *Recent Advances in the Study of Raptor Diseases*. Chiron Publications, Keighley.

PEIRCE, M. A. 1984A. Haematozoa of Zambian birds. I. General survey. *J. Nat. Hist.* **18**: 105–22.

PEIRCE, M. A. 1984B. Haematozoa of Zambian birds. XI. Observations on re-trapped birds. *Bull. Zambian Orn. Soc.* **16**: 10–12.

PEIRCE, M. A. & BEVAN, B. J. 1977. Blood parasites of imported psittacine birds. *Vet. Rec.* **100**: 282–5.

PEIRCE, M. A., CHEKE, A. S. & CHEKE, R. A. 1977. A survey of blood parasites of birds in the Mascarene Islands, Indian Ocean, with descriptions of two new species and taxonomic discussion. *Ibis* **119**: 451–61.

PEIRCE, M. A. & MARQUISS, M. 1983. Haematozoa of British birds. VII. Haematozoa of raptors in Scotland with a description of *Haemoproteus nisi* sp.nov. from the sparrowhawk (*Accipiter nisus*). *J. Nat. Hist.* **17**: 813–21.

PEIRCE, M. A. & MEAD, C. J. 1984. Haematozoa of British birds. VIII. Blood parasites of migrants, particularly the willow warbler *Phylloscopus trochilus*. *J. Nat. Hist.* **18**: 335–40.

WARNER, R. E. 1968. The role of introduced diseases in the extinction of the endemic Hawaiian avifauna. *Condor* **70**: 101–20.

DISEASE-RELATED ASPECTS OF CONSERVING THE ENDANGERED HAWAIIAN CROW

C. DAVID JENKINS[1], STANLEY A. TEMPLE[1], CHARLES VAN RIPER[2] & WALLACE R. HANSEN[3]

1 Department of Wildlife Ecology, University of Wisconsin, Madison, Wisconsin 53706, USA
2 Department of Wildlife and Fisheries, Biology and Co-operative Park Study Unit, University of California, Davis, California 95616, USA
3 National Wildlife Health Laboratory, U.S. Fish and Wildlife Service, Madison, Wisconsin 53711, USA

ABSTRACT

The Hawaiian Crow (*Corvus hawaiiensis*) is one of the most endangered endemic birds of the Hawaiian Islands. Its numbers have declined steadily during historical times, and fewer than 20 wild crows now survive in scattered areas of montane forest on the Kona coast of the island of Hawaii. One of the most obvious causes of the wild population's recent decline has been poor recruitment. We have found a high rate of infertility among eggs laid, a high rate of mortality among nestlings, and low initial survival of fledglings to be significant factors depressing recruitment. Exotic diseases, especially avian malaria and avian pox, seem to play central roles in these reproductive dysfunctions. Although habitat loss, persecution and disease have worked in concert to bring the crow to its present status, disease problems may be the single most important factor now preventing a population recovery.

INTRODUCTION

The Hawaiian Crow or Alala (*Corvus hawaiiensis*) is the only extant corvid inhabiting the Hawaiian Archipelago, although Olson & James (1982) reported fossil evidence of at least three additional *Corvus* species from the islands of Oahu and Molokai. Historically, the Alala has occurred only on the island of Hawaii, where it has recently been restricted primarily to the southwestern corner of the island (*Figure 1*). Within its range, the crow was once numerous (Henshaw 1902; Munro 1944; Perkins 1893, 1903; Wilson & Evans 1893). Since the early 1900s, however, numbers have declined drastically, and by the mid-1940s the bird had disappeared from lower altitudes of its former range (Banko & Banko 1980). The species now exists in disjunct and isolated subpopulations located within the higher elevation native forests of the North and South Kona Districts (*Figure 1*) and has become one of the most endangered of the endemic Hawaiian birds (King 1980; Burr *et al.* 1982). Scott *et al.* (1986) estimated during their 1978–80 censuses that there were only about 76 Hawaiian Crows left in the

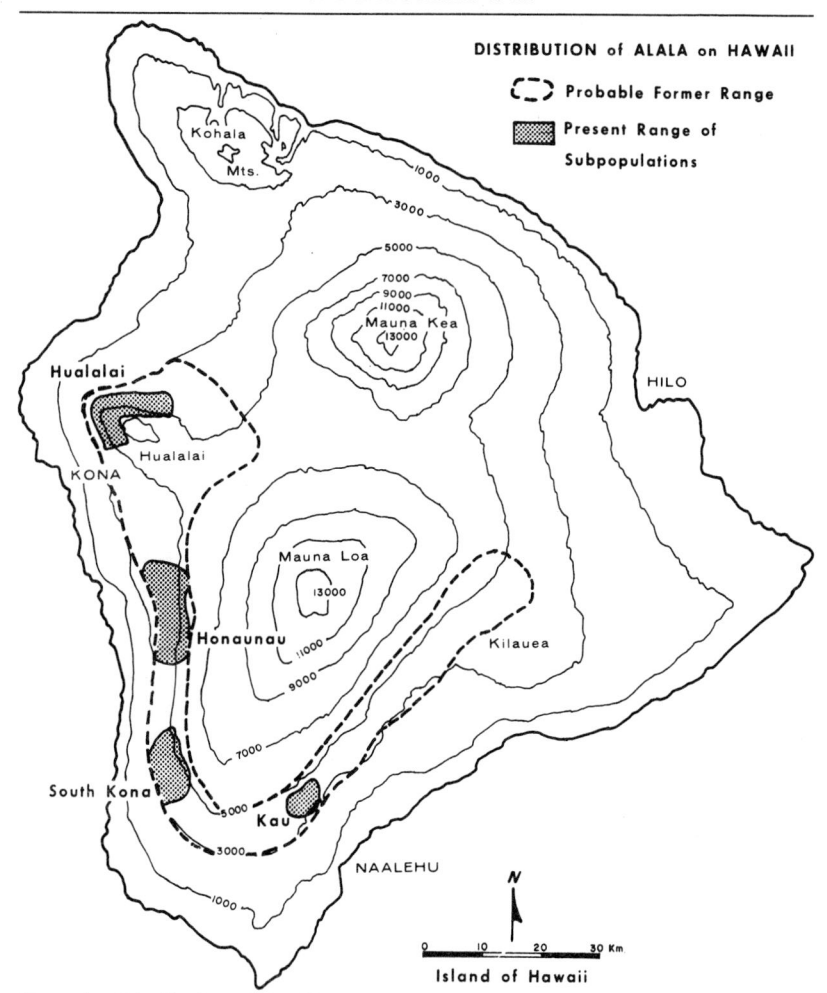

Figure 1: Distribution of the Hawaiian Crow or Alala (*Corvus hawaiiensis*) showing the probable former range of the species and the known ranges of the four existing subpopulations.

wild. However, more recent estimates suggest that by 1985 the population had declined to fewer than 12 birds (Scott & Kepler 1985; J. Giffin, pers. comm.). *Figure 2*, for example, plots the course of the recent decline of the Hualalai population.

Introduced diseases have been implicated as a factor in the decline of certain avian populations, particularly those that are small and isolated (Jackson 1978). Warner (1968) did preliminary work with mosquito-borne avian malaria and pox in Hawaii, and he suggested that the extinction or decline in numbers of many Hawaiian bird species was the direct result of these introduced diseases. More recent studies by van Riper *et al.* (1986) suggest that avian malaria was not a detriment to native Hawaiian birds until some time after 1920. At present, however, this introduced parasite is having a serious impact on native bird

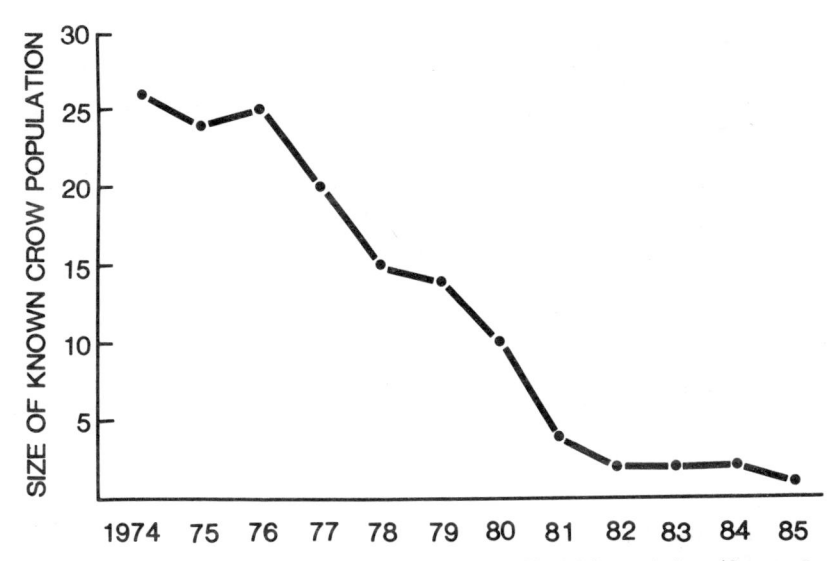

Figure 2: The recent decline in crow numbers in the Hualalai population. (*Source:* J. Giffin, 1983 and personal communication.)

populations, and is one of the major factors limiting endemic bird populations in the islands today (Ralph & van Riper 1985; Cooper, this volume).

During January–August 1979 and February–September 1980, we studied the Hawaiian Crow with the hope of understanding its continuing decline. In this paper we report the occurrence of avian malaria (*Plasmodium relictum capistranoae*) and avian pox (*Poxvirus avium*) in the Hawaiian Crow. We also discuss the impact that these two introduced diseases may be having on the Hawaiian Crow population.

STUDY AREA

We studied three disjunct breeding populations of Hawaiian Crows (*Figure 1*). The first, the Honaunau population, was located between 1200 and 1400 metres a.s.l. in the Honaunau Forest Reserve; the second, the South Kona population, was located between 1400m and 1500m on the McCandless Ranch. Both study sites were on the western slope of Mauna Loa. The third population, the Hualalai population, was located on the Puu Waawaa Ranch between 1500m and 1600m on the northwest slope of Hualalai. The nesting areas were primarily in mesic (moist), or wet, closed Ohia (*Metrosideros polymorpha*) forests with scattered emergent Koa (*Acacia koa*) in the higher elevations.

METHODS

At the end of each breeding season (July) we captured adult crows at their nesting sites (Sakai & Jenkins 1982). Each captured bird was measured and banded with U.S. Fish and Wildlife Service metal bands and an individual combination of coloured plastic bands. Hand-caught nestling and fledgling crows were also measured and banded. Before releasing birds, we prepared a thin blood smear from a clipped claw. Slides were air-dried, then immediately fixed for 30 seconds in absolute methanol. Blood slides were treated for 30 minutes with Giemsa stain in a solution buffered with Na_2PO_4 and K_2PO_4 to a pH of 7.17. Each slide was read under oil immersion at 1000× for 10 minutes, or until a minimum of 25,000 red blood cells (RBC) had been examined, as described by van Riper et al. (1986).

In 1980 we also obtained 1.0ml samples of whole blood from the brachial veins of captured crows for serum analysis. Whole blood samples were centrifuged at the end of each collection day. Serum was then frozen in cryotubes and later shipped in liquid nitrogen to the U.S. Fish and Wildlife National Wildlife Health Laboratory in Madison, Wisconsin. Sera from eight Hawaiian crows (three adults and five nestlings) were tested for precipitating antibodies to avipoxvirus in the Ouchterlony (1949) double immunodiffusion test. Diffusion plates were made with 1 percent Noble agar, 13 percent sodium chloride, and 0.01 percent Thimersal U.S.P. as described by Tripathy et al. (1970). The fowlpox virus strain ORT 101 obtained from the American Type Culture Collection (ATCC VR-228) and a poxvirus isolate 83-175 from a Hawaiian Amakihi (*Loxops virens virens*) were both used as antigens. Poxvirus antigens were prepared by homogenization of infected chorioallantoic membranes (CAM) of chicken-egg passage-three material. Thirty μl quantities of virus antigen or serum were added to each test well of the agar plate. A reference anti-fowlpox serum (Vineland strain) was used as a positive antibody control. Normal CAM was used as a negative antigen control. Plates were incubated in a moist chamber at room temperature and were examined for lines of identity, indicating the presence of poxvirus antibody, at 24 hours then periodically over a five-day period.

We carefully examined all captured birds and noted any pox-like lesions. We also monitored development of pox-like lesions on nestlings by examining films from time-lapse cameras mounted at selected nests.

Throughout each field season we monitored mosquito populations by regularly checking potential oviposition sites for evidence of mosquito larvae. Samples of all mosquito larvae were later identified in the laboratory. In addition, we analysed light-trap data provided by the Hawaii Department of Public Health to assess seasonal changes in adult mosquito populations in the Kona area.

RESULTS

During the two years of this study, 16 Hawaiian Crows were captured and examined. Four birds (two adults, two fledglings) were captured in the Hualalai study area, seven (two adults, five nestling or fledglings) in the Honaunau study area, and five (two adults, three nestling or fledglings) in the South Kona study area. Although our sample size seems small, the number of birds examined represented over 20 percent of the extant wild population.

Occurrence of avian malaria

We detected a heavy infection with avian malaria in one of the ten nestlings and fledglings that we examined. The malaria parasite was a member of the *Plasmodium relictum* group, and was undoubtedly *P. r. capistranoae*, the only known *Plasmodium* parasite in the islands (Laird & van Riper 1981). There were numerous multiple invasions of erythrocytes, with as many as eight merozoites penetrating a single erythrocyte. Prominent vacuolation was evident in developing schizonts, and up to three schizonts frequently reached maturity in the same cell. Gametocytes had conspicuous pigment granules scattered throughout the cytoplasm. The mature micro- and macrogametocytes averaged 7µm in diameter when spherical, and up to 8.5 × 5.5µm when oval; host cells were often enuculeate. Laird & van Riper (1981) described similar parasites in native birds on Mauna Loa, Hawaii. None of the six adult Hawaiian Crows that we bled had visible malaria parasites in their blood.

We inspected the nest that produced the malaria-infected young several times during the nestling period. Two recently hatched nestlings (less than two days old) were found in the nest when we first checked it. Twenty days later the nest contained only one nestling, which appeared healthy and weighed 320 grammes. We observed the remaining nestling being fed by its parents up to age 41 days. When the nestling was 48 days old, we again examined the nest contents because the nestling had not yet fledged. The mean fledging age for six apparently healthy Hawaiian Crow nestlings was 42.3 ± 1.2 days. The bird was weak and emaciated, weighing only 238 grammes. Mean fledging weight for all other crow nestlings was 452 ± 40 grammes. The nestling was unable to raise its head, and the nest was fouled with an accumulation of faeces because the bird was apparently too weak to defaecate over the nest rim. On this visit we took the blood sample which revealed the extremely high parasitaemia. The nestling was observed alive in the nest the following day. On our next visit to the nest site (when the nestling was 57 days old), we found the nestling fledged but unable to fly. Four days later the parents were still in the nesting area, but we were unable to locate the fledgling or its carcass. Young typically remain with their parents for nearly one year.

Occurrence of avian pox

We observed cutaneous lesions resembling those of avian pox on two of the ten Hawaiian Crow nestlings or fledglings that we examined. Both infected birds were from the same nest. On the time-lapse films, the first lesion was visible as a small pink dot just over the left eye of the smallest nestling 13 days before it fledged. A lesion was visible on the larger bird three days later, just over the right eye. Within five days, lesions were present on both sides of the face on both birds and increased in number and size throughout the remaining nestling period. In all other respects the nestlings behaved and developed normally when compared with apparently healthy birds.

We first examined the larger bird three days after it fledged, and the smaller bird on the day it left the nest. Each had several wart-like, cutaneous lesions surrounding both eyes, on the rictus (fleshy part of the edge of the mouth) and on the bill near the nares and the culmen (*Figure 3*). Some of the lesions, particularly on the rictus, were open and bleeding. The smaller bird had no claw on the fourth digit of its left foot. This bird also had four lesions on the right tarsus. Its sibling showed one lesion on the inside of the left carpus.

Following fledging, the bird that had lost a claw had some difficulty perching, and was always found closer to the ground than its sibling. We were able to capture and examine both fledglings repeatedly. During this period, some lesions began to dry and slough while others enlarged and became open and bleeding. On the seventh day after it fledged we could locate only the larger fledgling with its parents; two days later we could not locate either fledgling although we found both adults.

Precipitating antibodies against fowlpox virus ORT-101 were detected in five

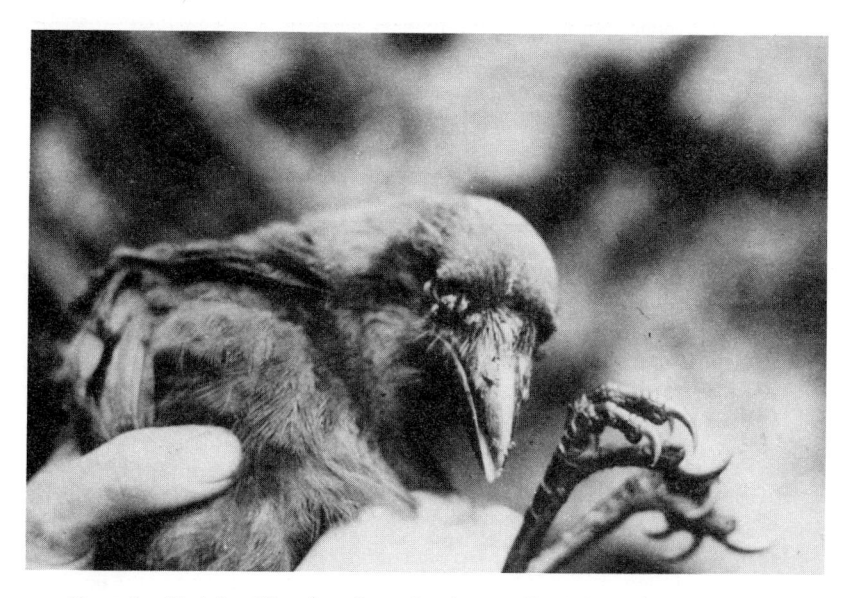

Figure 3: Fledgling Hawaiian Crow showing pox-like lesions. (*Photo*: Temple)

of eight Hawaiian Crow sera; all of the three sera from adults and two of the five from nestlings. Three of these positive sera, all from adults, also had lines of precipitation against the Hawaiian poxvirus isolate. Precipitating lines of identity were first formed for three Hawaiian Crow serum samples after 24 hours of incubation against both poxvirus test antigens. After 92 hours, two additional bands appeared for two more serum samples against the ORT-101 poxvirus antigen but not the Hawaiian poxvirus isolate. Lines of precipitation were better defined against the ORT-101 antigen, suggesting that there was a closer identity with that antigen.

Vector distributions

Light-trap data from Goff & van Riper (1980), and additional data obtained from the Vector Control Branch of the Hawaii Department of Public Health for the years 1972–82 show that the numbers of mosquitoes trapped during any month are generally quite low, and are highly variable from month to month. On average, however, mosquito numbers peak during the crow's breeding period (*Figure 4*).

Our larva and pupa surveys also substantiate this point. We found *Culex quinquefasciatus* larvae at elevations up to 1378 metres in the Honounnou Forest and up to 1470m on McCandless Ranch. During the months of April to July, larvae were found in transient pools, puddles, and small reservoirs, such as depressions in the trunks of fallen trees. We were, however, unable to locate any mosquito breeding sites in the study areas during February and March. This is much the same pattern that Goff & van Riper (1980) found in their study on Mauna Loa.

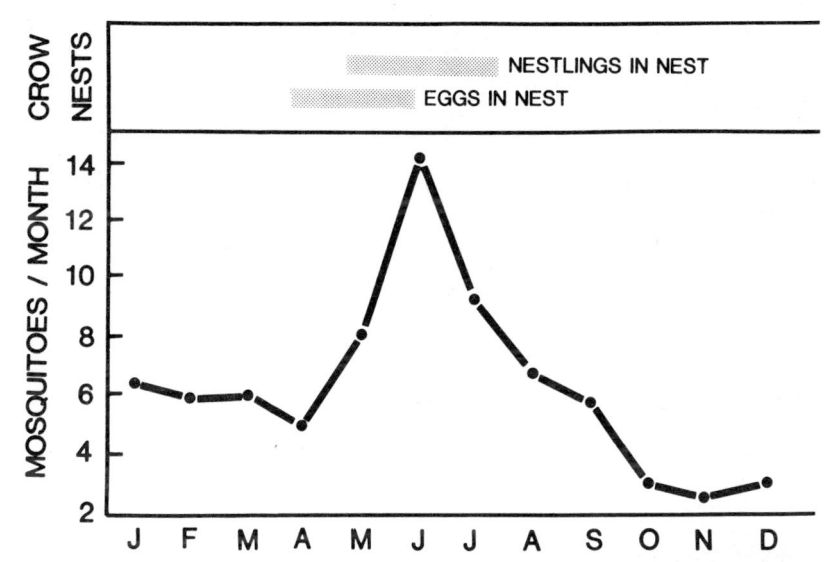

Figure 4: Annual cycles of mosquito numbers and Hawaiian Crow breeding activities. Mosquito data based on mean number of mosquitoes trapped in the Kona District per month, 1972–1982, by the Hawaiian Department of Public Health (personal communication).

DISCUSSION

Avian malaria in Hawaiian Crows

We have presented evidence here of the occurrence of avian malaria in the Hawaiian Crow population. A fair body of additional evidence from previous studies supports these findings.

In June 1970, W. Banko captured two fledglings from North Kona, one of which appeared anaemic (W. Banko, pers. comm.). Blood smears taken five days after capture were read by A. Miyahara of the University of Hawaii. He reported 'a moderate number of malarial parasites' from the smaller anaemic bird. The smear from the second bird contained 'a few malarial bodies'. Both birds were shipped to the Patuxent Wildlife Research Center on 4 August 1970, where the smaller one died shortly after arrival. Post-mortem examination revealed an enlarged spleen, and a liver impression showed an area 'suggestive of early malarial schizonts'. The second bird survived for three years at Patuxent in apparently good health but died suddenly in October 1973. The post-mortem examination revealed a very enlarged haemorrhagic spleen (10 × normal size) and an enlarged and friable liver. Although there was no sign of *Plasmodium* in any tissue, the condition of the spleen and liver suggests that some type of blood infection existed (J. Carpenter, pers. comm.).

In 1973 W. Banko (Banko & Banko 1980) discovered a nestling, near fledging age, dead in the nest. There were no visible external signs of disease. Unfortunately, the carcass was not recovered for further analysis. During the first year of our study we found the carcass of a fledgling beneath a nest. Post-mortem examination revealed an enlarged spleen and liver (J. Carpenter, pers. comm.).

Avian pox in Hawaiian Crows

We have also presented evidence of avian pox in the Hawaiian Crow population. The results of the immunodiffusion test indicate that both adult and fledgling Hawaiian Crows had antibodies to fowlpox virus. The early appearance of lines of identity for three of the sera suggests that the birds may have been infected recently or that they may have had multiple poxvirus exposures. However, the weak antibody reaction of sera from two fledgling crows with prominent 'poxvirus-like' cutaneous lesions suggests that the latter may be true, especially for the adult birds since they have not been seen with typical poxvirus lesions.

The reaction of the two Hawaiian Crow sera collected from the birds with numerous 'pox-like' lesions, probably relates to the sensitivity of the serological test used, but may also reflect the time following disease exposure that the serum sample was collected. Antibody production in the poxvirus infected birds may not have reached the threshold level required for detection by the immunodiffusion test. Therefore, some or all of the AGP negative crow sera may have had poxvirus antibody that was not detected by the test. Carpenter (1968) has indicated that the precipitation test is 1000 times less sensitive than a passive haemagglutination test for detecting antibody.

The stronger reaction of the Hawaiian Crow sera with the fowlpox antigen than the Hawaiian Amakihi poxvirus isolate may indicate the presence of more than one poxvirus strain on the island of Hawaii. This is not unusual since members of the fowlpox subgroup of avipoxviruses that infect canaries, sparrows, pigeons, etc. are distinct poxviruses, yet they show some serological cross-reactivity. The resolution of this question will require comparison of poxvirus field isolated from Hawaii.

In addition to being infected with malaria, the two fledglings brought in from captivity by Banko in 1970 had 'observable pox-like lesions on the bill and head' (J. Carpenter, pers. comm.). Giffin (1983) reports finding a fledgling with pox-like lesions in Honaunau Forest. This fledgling was produced by the same pair that produced the two pox-infected birds described in our study. Although Giffin tentatively diagnosed the disease as pox, it was not confirmed by isodiagnosis or electronmicroscopic tissue examination (Scullion, this volume).

The occurrence of pox in the crow does not appear to be a recent phenomenon. Ranchers (N. Greenwell & G. Schactauer, pers. comm.) report seeing young crows with visible lesions around the eyes. Perkins (1903) mentions the crow as one of the birds which was '. . . affected by a disease which caused swellings on the legs and feet as well as on the head at the base of the bill and on the skin around the eyes'.

Disease vectors on Hawaii

Laird & Van Riper (1981) demonstrated that *Culex quinquefasciatus* is the primary vector for *Plasmodium relictum* on Hawaii. This mosquito is probably the primary, but by no means only, vector for avian pox as well. Vectors of avian malaria and pox are present in sufficient numbers to spread diseases to susceptible hosts. Moreover, as *C. quinquefasciatus* is an ornithophilic mosquito, small vector numbers are capable of transmitting these diseases to highly susceptible Hawaiian birds, as van Riper *et al.* (1986) suggest happens in other forest areas on Mauna Loa.

Peak mosquito populations occur during the nestling and fledgling stages of the crows' breeding cycle. Young birds are especially vulnerable to biting mosquitoes due to their lack of defensive behaviour, and to their large areas of unfeathered epidermis (Blackmore & Dow 1958). In addition, juveniles are more likely than adults to succumb to malaria (Herman 1968).

The concurrence of peak mosquito numbers with the crow's breeding season occurs, in part, because of weather patterns. The region that the Hawaiian Crow occupies at present is somewhat anomalous in regard to rainfall patterns. When most regions of the islands are experiencing rain during the winter months, the Kona area is in its period of lowest rainfall. On the other hand, during the normally 'dry' summer period, the Kona area receives the bulk of its precipitation. Average monthly mosquito-trap totals from Kona (*Figure 4*) show that mosquito populations peak during the wettest months, April to October.

The principal breeding season for most native birds on the windward side of Hawaii is December to May (Berger 1981). Our observations suggest that on the west side of the island most birds nest later, principally from April to June. Circumstantial evidence is given by the proportion of passerine nestlings in the crow's diet which peaks during these months (Sakai *et al.* 1986). If, as has been shown in other birds, breeding activities induce a relapse of malarial infections (Beaudoin *et al.* 1971), a large reservoir of patently infected birds would exist concomitantly with the peak in mosquito populations. Warm temperatures at the time of the mosquito population's peak also probably enhance the completion of the *P. relictum* sexual cycle in the insect host, thus increasing the probability of successful transmission.

A diet containing a large proportion of fruits (Sakai *et al.* 1986), restricts the crow to mid-elevational ranges and thus places it in continuous contact with mosquitoes. In addition, there is some evidence that crows move to lower altitudes during the winter months (Giffin 1983) where mosquitoes are more likely to remain abundant.

Impact of disease on Hawaiian Crows

There is no conclusive evidence of Hawaiian Crow deaths resulting directly from an infection of avian malaria or pox. We have little doubt, however, that malaria and pox can cause direct mortality. Warner (1968) and van Riper *et al.* (1986) have demonstrated the susceptibility of many native Hawaiian birds to avian malaria. In van Riper's study, native birds were always more susceptible to malaria than were introduced species. Native birds exhibited a wide range of immunogenetic capability, apparently related to the populations' experience of the disease. Warner also documented mortality in captive wild Hawaiian birds suffering from a disease thought to be avian pox. Wright (1986) has shown a synergistic relationship between pox and malaria in wild turkeys (*Meleagris gallopavo*). Her findings suggest a greater likelihood of mortality in the birds that have both infections. The severity of both the malaria and pox infections we observed was great enough to make deaths likely, especially in young birds.

Increased susceptibility of infected crows to predation, starvation, and secondary infection is also a significant source of indirect mortality, especially in the case of avian pox. Healthy crow fledglings spend their first few days out of the nest very near the ground while they learn to fly. There they are susceptible to an array of introduced predators, especially the mongoose (*Herpestes auropunctatus*) and feral cat (*Felis catus*). A flightless fledgling weakened by malaria or with vision and mobility impaired by pox lesions would be particularly vulnerable to predation.

In addition to increasing susceptibility to predation, pox lesions around the eyes can interfere with the birds' ability to find food. Eruptions on the gape and bill may also impair feeding. Pox lesions which are open and bleeding provide prime sites for the introduction of secondary bacterial infections.

The presence of 'pox-like' lesions on two birds, together with the positive serological results, indicates that a high proportion of Hawaiian Crows are exposed to poxviruses during their lifetime. Since poxviruses are known to infect the young of several bird species, causing temporary but potentially debilitating lesions, this disease may be an important influence on the survivability of the Hawaiian Crow.

We can only speculate about the overall effect of disease on the dynamics of the crow population, but there are several reasons to suspect that the impact is great. Jenkins and Temple (unpublished data) have shown that poor recruitment—apparently resulting from infertility of eggs, poor hatchability, low nestling survival, and low post-fledging survival—is mainly responsible for the continuing decline of the Hawaiian Crow. Avian diseases may play an important role in several of these problems. During our study, at least four of ten nestlings and fledglings died from problems related to exotic diseases.

Regardless of whether or not avian diseases were initially responsible for the endangered status of the Hawaiian Crow, they are currently contributing to the population's continued decline, and present a serious impediment to its recovery. If recruitment remains low, there is little hope that the wild population will be able to maintain itself or increase. Captive breeding, as recommended in the Alala Recovery Plan (Burr *et al.* 1982; Burr 1984), may be the only hope for the short-term survival of the Hawaiian Crow.

ACKNOWLEDGEMENTS

We thank the trustees of Bishop Estate, William Rosehill, and William Stayton for allowing us access to Honaunau Forest and for their willingness to assist us. We are also grateful to Cynthia Sealy, manager and part owner of McCandless Ranch, who allowed us access to her property. The following individuals helped in various ways with field or laboratory work: Jon Giffin, Eleanor Brown and Nelson Santos. We are particularly thankful to Howard F. Sakai who assisted invaluably in all phases of this study. We also thank C. J. Ralph, Jim Jacobi and J. Michael Scott for their valuable advice and support. Our work was funded by the U.S. Forest Service, the U.S. National Park Service, the U.S. Fish and Wildlife Service, and the University of Wisconsin.

REFERENCES

BANKO, W. E. & BANKO, P. C. 1980. *CPSU/UH Avian History Report 6B. History of Endemic Hawaiian Birds. Part 1. Population Histories—Species Accounts. Forest Birds: Hawaiian Raven/Crow ('alala)*. Cooperative National Park Resources Studies Unit and University of Hawaii at Manoa.

BEAUDOIN, R. L., APPLEGATE, J. E., DAVIS, D. E. & McLEAN, R. G. 1971. A model for the ecology of avian malaria. *J. Wildl. Dis.* **7**: 5–13.

BERGER, A. J. 1981. *Hawaiian Birdlife*. 2nd edition. University Press of Hawaii, Honolulu.

BLACKMORE, J. S. & DOW, R. P. 1958. Differential feeding of *Culex tarsalis* on nestling and adult birds. *Mosq. News* **18(1)**: 15–18.

BURR, T. A., TOMICH, P. Q., KOSAKA, E., KRAMER, W., SCOTT, J. M., KRIDLER, E., GIFFIN, J., WOODSIDE, D. & BACHMAN, R. 1982. *Alala Recovery Plan*. U.S. Fish and Wildlife Service, Portland, Oregon.

BURR, T. A. 1984. *Alala Restoration Plan*. Dept. of Land and Natural Resources, Division of Forestry and Wildlife, Honolulu, Hawaii.

CARPENTER, P. L. 1968. *Immunology and Serology*. 2nd edition. W. B. Saunders, Philadelphia.

GIFFIN, J. G. 1983. *Final Report, 'Alala investigation. Pittman-Robertson Project No. W-18-R, Study No. R-II-B, 1976–1981*. State of Hawaii Dept. of Land and Natural Resources, Division of Forestry and Wildlife, Honolulu.

GOFF, M. L. & VAN RIPER, C. 1980. Distribution of mosquitoes (Diptera: Culicidae) on the east flank of Mauna Loa Volcano, Hawaii. *Pac. Insects* **22(1–2)**: 178–88.

HENSHAW, H. W. 1902. *Birds of the Hawaiian Islands, being a Complete List of the Birds of the Hawaiian Possessions with Notes on their Habits*. Thos. G. Thrum, Honolulu.

HERMAN, C. M. 1968. Blood protozoa of free-living birds. *Symp. Zool. Soc. Lond.* **24**: 177–95.

JACKSON, J. A. 1978. Alleviating problems of competition, predation, parasitism, and disease in endangered birds. *In:* Temple, S. A. (ed.). *Endangered Birds: Management Techniques for Preserving Threatened Species:* University of Wisconsin Press, Madison.

KING, W. B. 1980. *Endangered Birds of the World: The ICBP Red Data Book*. Smithsonian Institution Press, Washington, DC.

LAIRD, M. & VAN RIPER, C. 1981. Questionable reports of *Plasmodium* from birds in Hawaii, with recognition of *P. relictum* ssp. *capistranoae* (Russell, 1932) as the avian malaria parasite there. *In:* Canning, E. U. (ed.). *Parasitological Topics*, Special Publication No. 1, Allen Press, Lawrence, Kansas.

MUNRO, G. C. 1944. *Birds of Hawaii*. Tongg Publishing Co., Honolulu.

OLSON, S. L. & JAMES, H. F. 1982. *Prodromus of Fossil Avifauna of the Hawaiian Islands*. Smithsonian Contributions to Zoology 365. Smithsonian Inst. Press, Washington, DC.

OUCHTERLONY, O. 1949. Antigen-antibody reaction in gels. *Acta. Pathol. Microbiol. Scand.* **26**: 507–15.

PERKINS, R. C. L. 1893. Notes on collecting in Kona, Hawaii. *Ibis* **5**: 101–12.

PERKINS, R. C. L. 1903. *Fauna Hawaiiensis, 1(VI). Vertebrata*. Cambridge University Press.

RALPH, C. J. & VAN RIPER, C. 1985. Historical and current factors affecting Hawaiian native birds. *In:* Temple, S. A. (ed.). *Bird Conservation 2:* University of Wisconsin Press, Madison.

SAKAI, H. F. & JENKINS, C. D. 1982. Capturing the endangered Hawaiian Crow with mist nets. *N. Am. Bird Band.* **8(2)**: 54–5.

SAKAI, H. F., RALPH, C. J. & JENKINS, C. D. 1986. Foraging ecology of the Hawaiian Crow, an endangered generalist. *Condor* **88**: 211–19.

SCOTT, J. M. & KEPLER, C. B. 1985. Distribution and abundance of Hawaiian native birds: a status report. *In:* Temple, S. A. (ed.). *Bird Conservation 2:* University of Wisconsin Press, Madison.

SCOTT, J. M., MOUNTAINSPRING, S., RAMSEY, F. L. & KEPLER, C. B. 1986. Forest bird communities of the Hawaiian Islands: their dynamics, ecology, and conservation. *Studies in Avian Biology* **9**: 1–100.

TRIPATHY, D. N., HANSON, L. E. & MYERS, W. L. 1970. Passive hemagglutination test with fowlpox virus. *Avian Dis.* **14**: 29–38.

VAN RIPER, C., VAN RIPER, S. G., GOFF, M. L. & LAIRD, M. 1986. The epizootiology and ecological significance of malaria on the birds of Hawaii. *Ecological Monographs* **56**: 327–44.

WARNER, R. E. 1968. The role of introduced diseases in the extinction of the endemic Hawaiian avifauna. *Condor* **70**: 101–20.

WILSON, S. B. & EVANS, A. H. 1893. *Aves Hawaiiensis: The Birds of the Sandwich Islands, Part IV*. R. H. Porter, London.

WRIGHT, E. L. 1986. Interactive effects of turkey pox and malaria (*Plasmodium hermani*) on turkey poults. Master's Thesis, University of Florida, Gainesville, Florida.

MORTALITY, MORBIDITY AND BREEDING SUCCESS OF THE PINK PIGEON (*COLUMBA (NESOENAS) MAYERI*)

CARL G. JONES, DAVID M. TODD & YOUSOOF MUNGROO

Forestry Quarters, Black River, Mauritius

ABSTRACT

The Pink Pigeon is a highly endangered species with a wild population of fewer than 30 individuals. Captive populations have been established, and the two main ones are at the Government Aviaries in Black River, Mauritius, and the Jersey Wildlife Preservation Trust. In these two collections, 1447 eggs were laid between 1977 and 1986. Only about 732 (50.6 percent) were fertile, of which 370 (50.5 percent) hatched. Of these, 200 (54 percent) reached 30 days; 63.2 percent of fledglings survive to reach one year. The various factors that may contribute to these high mortality rates are appraised. Breeding success among the wild (free-living) Pink Pigeons is very low, and fewer than 10 percent of nests succeed in fledging any young.

Inbreeding is suspected to be depressing the breeding results of the captive birds and elevating the rates of mortality. The nesting failures of the wild pigeons are primarily due to egg predation.

Careful long-term management of both the wild and the captive populations will be essential in order to avoid the species' extinction.

INTRODUCTION

The Pink Pigeon (*Columba (Nesoenas) mayeri*), which is endemic to the island of Mauritius in the western Indian Ocean, has been the subject of a captive breeding programme for ten years. Since the first three were caught in March 1976 (McKelvey 1976), nearly 200 Pink Pigeons have been fledged at the Government Aviaries at Black River, Mauritius, and at the Jersey Wildlife Preservation Trust (JWPT). Captive-bred birds from these two collections have been used to establish four other breeding populations. Practical details of the captive breeding programme are given by Jones *et al.* (1983). In 1984/5, 22 Pink Pigeons bred in captivity were released into the botanical garden at Pamplemousses, Mauritius, to test the feasibility of a more ambitious release into an area of native forest (Todd 1984). The wild population has meanwhile apparently stabilized and now numbers about 20 birds.

Despite the success of the captive breeding programme, there is cause for concern because of the low rate of successful breeding, the incidence of developmental defects, and the relatively high mortality among sub-adult birds. A

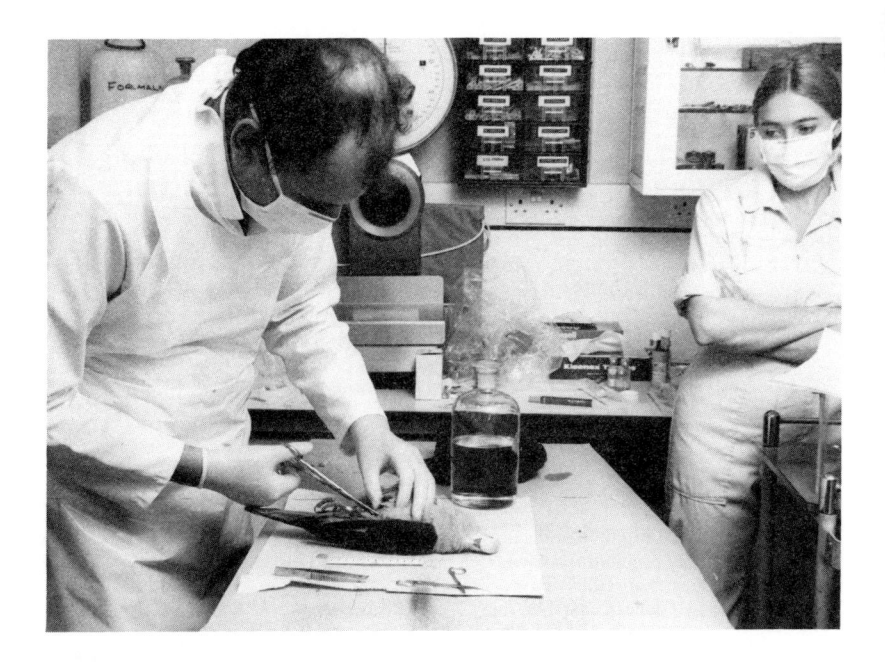

Figure 1: Post mortem examination of a Pink Pigeon (*Columba mayeri*). In recent years the species has been the subject of detailed clinical and pathological investigation, both on Mauritius and at the Jersey Wildlife Preservation Trust. (*Photo*: J. E. Cooper)

preliminary analysis of the breeding records and mortality data is presented here.

SOURCES OF DATA

Detailed records of the fate of all breeding attempts at the Government Aviaries and at the JWPT have been kept since the start of the captive breeding programme. Most of the Pink Pigeons that have died in captivity have been referred to John E. Cooper at the Royal College of Surgeons of England, where they have been examined post mortem (*Figures 1* and *2*). Others have been examined at the JWPT. Although the resulting data have not yet been fully analysed, use has been made of early findings. Relevant information from studies of the wild Pink Pigeons and those released at Pamplemousses are also discussed.

FINDINGS

MORTALITY OF JUVENILE AND ADULT PINK PIGEONS

More than a quarter of Pink Pigeons fledged at the Government Aviaries and the JWPT have failed to survive their first year. Mortality was relatively high

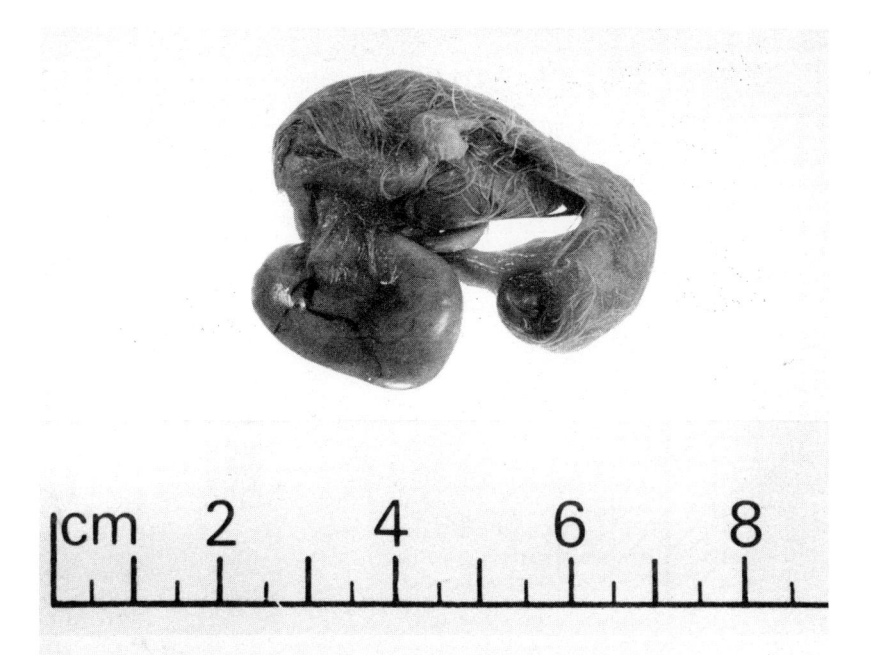

Figure 2: Embryos are examined carefully for developmental abnormalities as well as for the presence of infectious disease. The cause of death of this Pink Pigeon embryo was probably chilling. (*Photo*: J. E. Cooper)

during the first two months of independent life, but then dropped markedly (*Figure 3*). Many of the deaths during the second six months of life were the result of emaciation following increased intraspecific aggression in the aviaries holding groups of young birds (see below). *Figure 4* shows the age distribution of deaths in subsequent years. The maximum life span so far recorded is for a male trapped as an adult in 1976, which is still alive in its thirteenth year of captivity. Although a female trapped as an adult in 1977 also survives, female Pink Pigeons have tended not to live as long as males. Because wild-caught pigeons and members of each annual cohort of captive-bred birds still survive, it is impossible to calculate mean life spans accurately for males and females that live for more than one year. However, if only those pigeons hatched before 1 January 1981 are considered, and it is assumed that wild birds trapped as adults were one year old when caught, minimum mean life spans of 6.6 years for males and 5.2 years for females are obtained. The shorter lives of females may be in part a result of management aimed at maximizing egg production. The Pink Pigeons at JWPT live longer on average than those at the Government Aviaries and there is therefore a greater proportion of older birds in that population (*Figure 5*).

Factors associated with the deaths of fledged Pink Pigeons at the Government Aviaries and the JWPT, and those that were culled or died in quarantine at the Royal College of Surgeons, are shown in *Table 1*. In nearly 30 percent of cases there was no apparent cause of death. Thirty-five percent of deaths could be

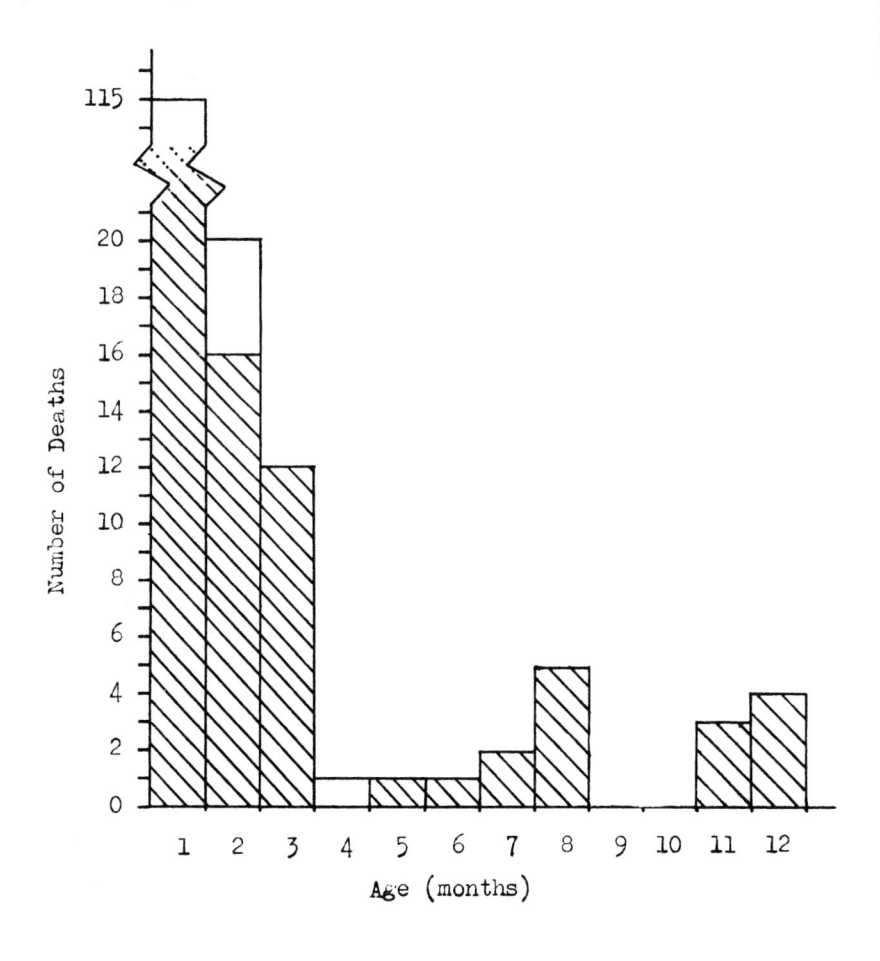

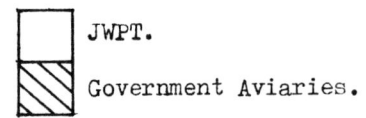

Figure 3: Age distribution of deaths of Pink Pigeons in their first year, at the Government Aviaries and at the Jersey Wildlife Preservation Trust.

attributed to nutritional or developmental defects, though many of the pigeons dying in an emaciated condition were the victims of intraspecific aggression. Infectious diseases were diagnosed as the cause of only ten deaths (12.7 percent), while faulty management and accidents accounted for more than 20 percent of the total.

Little is known of the life expectancy and mortality of adult Pink Pigeons in the wild. It has been suggested that feral cats (*Felis catus*) and mongooses (*Herpestes auropunctatus*) might kill some birds forced to feed on the ground by seasonal

Figure 4: Age distribution of deaths of Pink Pigeons, post fledging, at the Government Aviaries and at the Jersey Wildlife Preservation Trust.

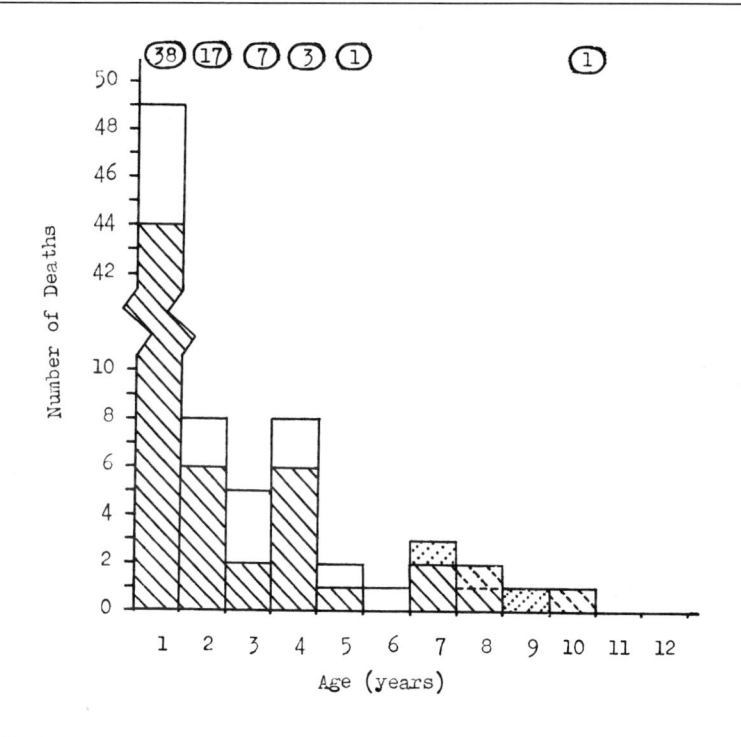

food shortages (Jones 1987). McKelvey (1976) reported an attack on a Pink Pigeon by a Peregrine Falcon (*Falco peregrinus*), but this must be a very rare occurrence as there have been only two other records of Peregrine Falcons on Mauritius. Pink Pigeons are killed during cyclones, or starve later because the trees have been stripped of fruits, flowers and leaves, but cyclones hit Mauritius on average only once every four years, and even then the Pink Pigeon habitat is not always adversely affected (Jones 1987). Because of its reputation for being poisonous, the Pink Pigeon has never apparently been hunted on a large scale, but birds have occasionally been shot in the past (Jones 1987). However, of the 22 Pink Pigeons released in Pamplemousses, up to 15 were killed or injured by intruders with catapults. Since 1976, eleven adult Pink Pigeons have been trapped for the captive breeding programme.

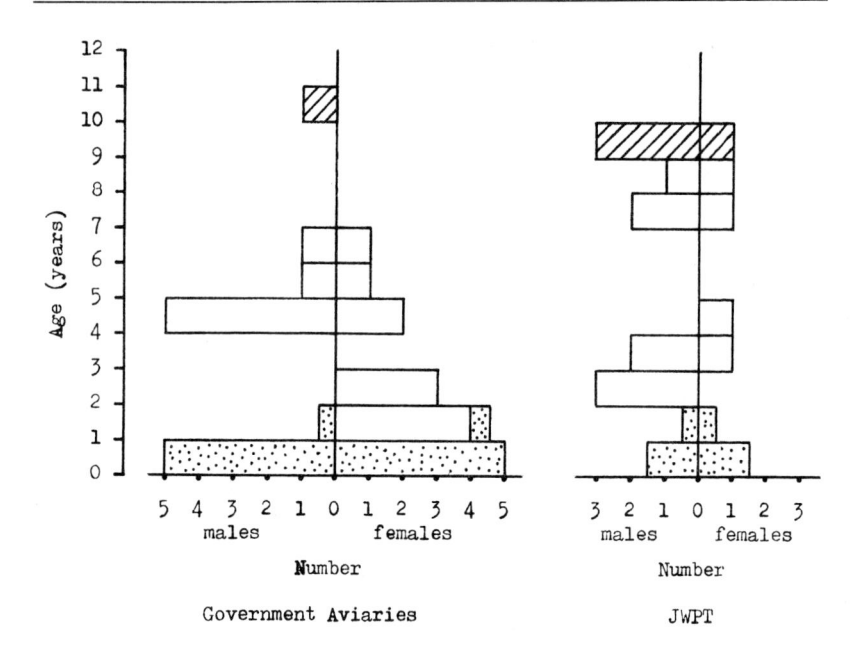

Unsexed.

Minimum ages of pigeons trapped as adults.

Figure 5: Age structure of the captive Pink Pigeon populations at the Government Aviaries and the Jersey Wildlife Preservation Trust on 31 December 1985.

NUTRITIONAL DISEASES

In the wild, Pink Pigeons eat the leaves, buds, flowers, fruit and seeds of a range of native and exotic plant species, and have also been reported to eat animals such as snails and tadpoles (Jones 1987). At the Government Aviaries, they are fed on a variety of grains and pulses obtained locally, and the birds supplement this diet with leaves and shoots from the trees growing in their aviaries. Due to local shortages, it has not always proved possible to maintain a varied diet, and as a result some pigeons have developed conditions caused by vitamin deficiencies.

Young Pink Pigeons fed on diets with a high proportion of millet have tended to grow slowly and to have a ragged appearance. The growing feathers sometimes lack pigment, and in severe cases debris accumulates in the corner of the gape, the eyelid margins become granulated, and an exudate causes them to stick together. These are signs of a pantothenic acid deficiency but hypovitaminosis A is also a possibility (Arnall & Keymer 1975; Scott *et al.* 1982). The condition is not expressed equally in all squabs fed on the same diet, and some do not appear to be affected at all. This suggests that some birds are genetically more susceptible to a shortage than others.

Juvenile Pink Pigeons kept without access to fresh leaves develop signs

Table 1: Causes of mortality of fledged Pink Pigeons at the Government Aviaries, the JWPT, and the Royal College of Surgeons (RCS).

Proximate or Contributory Causes	Govt. Aviaries	JWPT	RCS	Total No.	%
Unknown/Unidentified	17	6	0	23	29.1
Nutritional and developmental problems	19	2	7	28	35.4
Culled (leg deformities)	0	2	5		
Culled (cerebellar hypoplasia)	0	0	1		
Emaciated	5	0	1		
Emaciated/vitamin A deficiency	6	0	0		
Pantothenic acid deficiency	1	0	0		
Culled (perosis)	1	0	0		
Opisthotonus/fits	4	0	0		
Ataxia	1	0	0		
Articular gout	1	0	0		
Management and accidents	10	8	0	18	22.8
'Stress'	2	0	0		
Aortic rupture	1	0	0		
Circulatory failure	0	1	0		
Impaction of colon	1	0	0		
Gut stasis	0	1	0		
Self-mutilation	0	1	0		
Accident	0	1	0		
Infection following head injury	1	0	0		
Entangled in creeper	2	0	0		
Escaped	0	2	0		
Ruptured crop	1	0	0		
Haemorrhage post-vaccination	0	1	0		
Accidental overdose	1	0	0		
Culled (permanent luxation)	0	1	0		
Culled (fractures)	1	0	0		
Infectious disease	9	0	1	10	12.7
Unconfirmed Newcastle disease	4	0	0		
Diphtheritic cloacitis	2	0	0		
Unconfirmed coccidiosis	2	0	0		
Caseous air sacculitis	0	0	1		
Necrotic lesions in the liver	1	0	0		
TOTAL	55	16	8	79	

characteristic or suggestive of a vitamin A deficiency. These included the appearance of small white pustules in the buccal cavity and a watery discharge from the nostrils and eyes. In one case deposition of urates on the heart was noted post mortem, probably indicative of renal failure, possibly exacerbated by vitamin A deficiency. One young pigeon showing signs of vitamin A deficiency suffered fits and died in opisthotonus, and another had poor coordination and balance. When this second bird was culled as an adult, it was found to have cerebellar hypoplasia (Cooper *et al.* 1987). A squab which trembled continuously and had problems balancing died at the age of 14 days. Six Pink Pigeon squabs at the Government Aviaries had what appeared to be 'clubbed down' on hatching, usually a sign of riboflavin or zinc deficiency (Scott *et al.* 1982). The six were the offspring of one pair, and it is possible that a genetic defect inhibiting the assimilation of this vitamin was involved.

SKELETAL DEFECTS

'Inclined feet' has been a common skeletal defect in the captive Pink Pigeon populations. It has been noted in 18 pigeons at the Government Aviaries and one at JWPT. This condition expresses itself as an inward twisting of one or both feet, and first becomes noticeable when the young pigeon is about two weeks old. A mild case is difficult to detect and the bird is able to perch normally. However, in its severest form the feet are so badly twisted that the bird has to balance on its metatarso-phalangeal joints. It has not proved possible to correct the deformity by the application of splints to the birds' legs and feet.

Three Pink Pigeon squabs bred at the Government Aviaries have sustained numerous fractures with no apparent history of trauma. One of these died before fledging, but with intensive care the other two survived. All three were closely related, two of them siblings, so this condition may be genetic in origin.

Several Pink Pigeon squabs developed 'slipped wing', which occurs when the carpus is rotated outwards by the weight of the growing primaries. 'Splayed legs' has affected at least 12 squabs at the Government Aviaries. It develops if the legs are forced apart as the body rapidly gains weight. The incidence of 'slipped wing' was found to be higher in inbred Giant Canadian Geese (*Branta canadensis maxima*) than in outbred ones (Kreeger & Walser 1984), while 'splayed legs' is particularly common in some inbred strains of falcons. There may, therefore, be a genetic component to both these conditions.

Cooper *et al.* (1987) found that three out of six Pink Pigeons examined had bent sterna. This condition, which may affect a quarter of all captive-bred pigeons on Mauritius, involves the buckling of the sternal carina and varies from a barely discernible wave to a marked kink. Affected birds show no obvious disability.

VIRAL, BACTERIAL AND PARASITIC INFECTIONS

The only blood parasite so far identified in Pink Pigeons is *Leucocytozoon marchouxi* (Peirce *et al.* 1977). This species had previously been recorded from two other columbiforms on Mauritius, the introduced Spotted Dove (*Streptopelia chinensis*) and the Barred Ground Dove (*Geopelia striata*) (Peirce *et al.* 1977). The results from the screening of Pink Pigeon blood samples for parasites are summarized in *Table 2*. It is striking that *Leucocytozoon* was found in samples from six out of seven Pink Pigeons awaiting release at Pamplemousses, but that none of the five already released was infected. It is possible that the birds in the release aviary were more stressed and so had a demonstrable parasitaemia. One of the six infected birds survived in the botanical garden for two years after release. A body detected in a lymphocyte from one of the released birds could not be identified.

Coccidial oocysts and an ascarid egg were isolated from the intestinal contents of one of two Pink Pigeons culled at the JWPT (Flach 1984). Three Pink Pigeons have died at the Government Aviaries showing signs of coccidiosis, but the Government's Animal Health Laboratory failed to confirm this diagnosis. Three others examined post mortem at the Royal College of Surgeons showed a diphtheritic cloacitis, which was suspected to be due to *Trichomonas gallinae* (J. E. Cooper, unpublished data). One squab at the JWPT has died of trichomoniasis, and McKelvey (1976) noted the death of a squab with the same disease.

Table 2: Results of examinations of blood samples from Pink Pigeons for parasites.

No. examined	Origin	No. infected	Species	Reference
6	Government Aviaries	0	—	Cooper et al (in press)
2	Government Aviaries	0	—	J. E. Cooper (pers. comm.)
4	?	1	*Leucocytozoon marchouxi*	Peirce (1984)
5	Pamplemousses (free)	1	unidentified	J. E. Cooper (pers. comm.)
7	Pamplemousses (caged)	6	*L. marchouxi*	J. E. Cooper (pers. comm.)
2	JWPT	0	—	Flach (1984)
7	Government Aviaries	0	—	Animal Health Laboratory, Mauritius

Table 3: Additional records of potentially pathogenic bacteria recorded from Pink Pigeons from the Government Aviaries.

Date	No. examined	Tissued examined	Species identified	Source
Jul '80	1	liver	*Pasteurella multocida*	AHL
Jul '80	1	liver, lung & exudate	*Aerobacter aerogenes* / *Streptococcus* sp.	AHL
May '81	1	liver	*Pasteurella gallinarum*	AHL
Aug '81	2	cloacal swab	*Salmonella typhimurium*	J. E. Cooper
Sept '81	1	liver / throat swab / faeces	*Staphylococcus* sp. / *Corynebacterium* sp. / *Staphylococcus* sp. / *Escherichia coli*	AHL
Dec '81	1	cloacal swab	Coccobacillus	AHL
Jul '82	1	liver	*Corynebacterium* sp.	AHL

Note: AHL = Animal Health Laboratory, Mauritius.

There have been no records of trichomoniasis in the wild population, but the young from two nests at Pamplemousses are thought to have died from this disease. The females from both nests, which failed within two days of each other, were found with their pharynges virtually blocked by 'canker' two weeks later. Following the observation of flagellates (Reece, this volume) from buccal swabs, both pigeons were treated and made full recoveries.

Cooper *et al.* (1987) listed bacterial and fungal species isolated from throat and gut swabs from six Pink Pigeons originating from the Government Aviaries. Some of those identified are potential avian pathogens, for example *Pasteurella* spp., *Yersinia* sp. and *Aspergillus* spp. Table 3 summarizes other records of bacteria isolated from Pink Pigeons. Bacterial infections that have been identified as a cause of death include one case involving a *Corynebacterium* sp. and two cases of coliform infection at the JWPT. Pneumonia was identified as the cause of death of one, possibly two, squabs at the JWPT and of one adult at the Rio Grande Zoological Park at Albuquerque, New Mexico.

None of the six pigeons culled at the Royal College of Surgeons in 1983 showed serum antibodies to Newcastle disease virus (paramyxoviruses 2–9, excluding 5) or to *Chlamydia psittaci* (Cooper *et al.* 1987). However, four Pink Pigeons which died in convulsions in 1985 were thought by Mauritius Government veterinary staff to have been suffering from Newcastle disease. At Albuquerque, four squabs died from *Herpesvirus* infections. This virus was found to be enzootic, though previously undetected, in the flock of Domestic Pigeons from which the foster-parents for Pink Pigeon eggs were drawn (Snyder *et al.* 1985).

Apart from the three squabs killed by maggots of the Tropical Nest Fly (*Passeromyia heterochaeta*), there is no evidence that insect parasites have caused any deaths, though it is probable that they act as vectors for some infections. A hippoboscid (*Ornithoctora plicata*) has been found on a Pink Pigeon squab in the wild and on adults at Pamplemousses. Simuliid flies are the normal vectors of *Leucocytozoon* species (Peirce *et al.* 1977), so it is possible that *Simulium ruficorne*, the only species recorded in Mauritius, feeds on the Pink Pigeon. Although suitable vectors for avian malaria are present, neither these parasites nor microfilariae have yet been identified in blood samples from Pink Pigeons. Pink Pigeons kept at Casela Bird Park in Mauritius, where a wide selection of

Table 4: The breeding success of Pink Pigeons at the Government Aviaries and the JWPT, contrasted with that reported for Domestic Pigeons.

| | Pink Pigeons |||| Domestic Pigeons |
| | Mauritius 1977–86 || Jersey 1977–86 || USA |
	No.	%	No.	%	%
No. of eggs	973		474		
No. (%) smashed	186	19.1	116/340	34.1	0 (?)
No. (%) fertile	415/742	55.9	101/254	39.8	82.4–88.3
Est. no. of fertile, unsmashed eggs	440		124		
No. (%) hatched	282	68.0	88	71.0	94.5–96.7
No. (%) fledged (30 days)	165	58.5	35	39.8	75.7–93.1
No. (%) to one year	96/158	60.8	26	74.3	
% of eggs fledged		17.0		7.4	60.2–79.1

Notes: Data for the Domestic Pigeon are from four years of the New Jersey Squab Breeding Contest and one year at the Chaffey Squab Breeding Experimental Station Contest (reviewed in Levi 1978). Data for the Pink Pigeon are from Jones *et al.* (1983), summaries in the journal *Dodo* 1977–1986 and unpublished information.

exotic species is on display, have been found infested with feather lice. These have not yet been identified.

'ADRENAL STRESS'

At the Government Aviaries, groups of juvenile Pink Pigeons are housed together to avoid socialization problems. However, if the groups are maintained for too long, the birds develop a dominance hierarchy (McKelvey 1976) and the subordinate birds may be continually harassed by the others. They then feed less or stop feeding altogether, rapidly lose weight, and may die from a variety of causes if they are not separated from the other birds (Jones *et al.* 1983). If a pair of adults is placed in an aviary, one of the birds, usually the female, may suffer in a similar manner if the pair proves incompatible. This can also happen with well-established pairs if only one bird is in breeding condition. As an example, a female placed in an aviary with a prospective mate was chased by the male, being frequently displaced from her perch. Although still outwardly healthy, she stopped feeding and lost 135g, 38 percent of her original weight, within 15 days. She was removed, and had to be hand-fed until strong enough to fend for herself. This condition is similar to that described as adrenal stress in Wood Pigeons (*Columba palumbus*) (see below).

BREEDING SUCCESS

Pink Pigeons had laid 973 eggs at the Government Aviaries and 474 at the JWPT by the end of 1986. Fertility was low when compared with that reported for the Domestic Pigeon (*Columba livia*) in the USA (Levi 1978) (*Table 4*), as was the hatchability of fertile, unbroken eggs and the proportion of squabs successfully fledged.

The limited data on wild Pink Pigeons suggest that they are no more successful at breeding than the captive ones, with less than 10 percent of the eggs surviving

Table 5: Rates of fledging and nest predation of wild Pink Pigeons compared with those of some other pigeon and dove species.

Species	No. of eggs	No. fledged	% eggs fledged	Overall % predation eggs	squabs
Pink Pigeon *Columba* (*Nesoenas*) *mayeri*—Mauritius	21–21	1	c. 4–5	(≤96)	
	51–27	7	c.12–14	71–82	0
	72–84	4	c. 5	c.80–95	
	100–120	≤8	≤7–8	(≤92)	
Feral Pigeon *C.livia*—England	812	384	47.3	18.7	c.5.4
Stock Dove *C.oenas*—Belgium	360	136	37.8	19.0	c.5.3
Wood Pigeon *C.palumbus*—England	1704	c.527	30.9	55.2	(≤11.2)
Collared Dove *Streptopelia decaocto*—Czechoslovakia	436	c.299	68.6	(≤2.8)	c.3.7
Turtle Dove *S.turtur*—England	621	c.242	39	34	(≤8)
Laughing Dove *S.senegalensis*—USSR	84	41	48.8	(≤28.6)	(≤17.8)
Ruddy Ground Dove *Columbina talpacoti*—Costa Rica	40	8	20.0	(≤50)	(≤30)
Cold-billed Ground Dove *C.cruziana*—Ecuador	477	c.263	55.2	(≤23.3)	(≤21.5)

Notes: Data for the Pink Pigeon are from McKelvey (1976, 1977), Temple (1978) and Jones (1987); where necessary the numbers of eggs have been estimated by assuming 1.5 to 1.75 eggs per clutch. Data for the other species are from Cramp (1985) and Ricklefs (1969) who refer to various original sources.

to produce fledged young. However, the main cause of failure is predation, which possibly accounts for the loss of at least 80 percent of all clutches (*Table 5*). Other known causes of failure in the wild are infertility and the destruction of nests during cyclones.

In the botanical garden at Pamplemousses, possibly as many as five out of nine nesting attempts failed due to predation by Common Mynahs (*Acridotheres tristis*), an introduced species common in the man-modified habitats but rare in the remnants of native forest. Apart from the eggs and squabs taken for the captive breeding programme, only one clutch of eggs is known to have been collected by humans and this is now in the Mauritius Institute (Jones *et al.* 1983).

Egg breakage

Captive Pink Pigeons tend to be clumsy on the nest and many eggs have been found cracked, dented or smashed. Eggs have also been pushed out of nests, often due to over-zealous incubation behaviour, for example when both parents try to sit at the same time. At the Government Aviaries, over a third of eggs left under Pink Pigeons have been damaged during the course of incubation (*Table 6*). This is partly due to inexperience; birds in their first year of laying at the JWPT broke 26 out of 58 eggs (44.8 percent), whereas those in their fourth year broke nine out of 44 (20.5 percent) (Rankine 1983). The difference is statistically significant ($X^2 = 5.557$, $P < 0.05$). In part to minimize such losses, both the Government Aviaries and the JWPT now foster eggs, under Barbary Doves (*Streptopelia 'risoria'*) on Mauritius and under doves and Domestic Pigeons in Jersey. The use of foster parents also enables the Pink Pigeon pairs

Table 6: Survival of Pink Pigeon eggs incubated by Pink Pigeons and by Barbary Doves at the Government Aviaries.

	Incubated by Pink Pigeons No.	%	Incubated by Barbary Doves No.	%	n	χ^2	P
No. of eggs	85		501				
No. (%) smashed	30	35.3	14	2.8	586	105.9	<0.001
No. (%) fertile	33/63	52.4	296/466	63.5	529	2.474	n.s.
Est. no. of fertile, unsmashed eggs	29		309				
No. (%) hatched	19	65.5	222	71.8	338	0.256	n.s.
No. (%) fledged	9	47.4	133	59.9	241	0.678	n.s.
No. (%) to one year	6	66.7	97	72.9	142	—	n.s.

to recycle more rapidly and so increases the production of eggs. The results obtained suggest that Barbary Doves are at least as successful at hatching Pink Pigeon eggs and raising the squabs as the Pink Pigeons themselves (*Table 6*). Fostering at the Government Aviaries has reduced the incidence of damage and displacement from the nest during incubation, but there is still appreciable loss (19 percent) during the first few hours before the eggs can be transferred. These losses include eggs laid directly off a perch. Rankine (1983) records thin and soft-shelled eggs at the JWPT and eleven eggs with very poor quality shells have been noted at the Government Aviaries, despite suitable sources of calcium being available.

The loss of eggs due to breakage in the nest appears to be rare in Domestic Pigeons, and it has never been recorded for wild free-living Pink Pigeons. It may have been the cause of one nest failure at Pamplemousses (Todd 1984), but predation could not be ruled out in that case.

Infertility

The percentage of infertile eggs laid by Pink Pigeons is about three times that found in Domestic Pigeons (*Table 4*). Preliminary findings suggest that inexperience and senility play a part, but they cannot account for the majority of infertile eggs. Rankine (1983) considered that failure to copulate successfully was a major cause of infertility, but this was difficult to substantiate. Spermatozoa from a testis smear examined in 1984 at the JWPT showed a number of abnormalities (J. E. Cooper, unpublished). It is not known whether other males are similarly affected. The presence of such abnormalities could account for the effect of inbreeding on fertility. Of 46 eggs laid by pairs including a bird with an inbreeding coefficient of 0.25, only 41.2 percent proved fertile. In contrast, the percentage of fertile eggs laid by brother-sister pairs or their equivalent kinship (kinship coefficient = 0.25) has been higher, though not significantly higher, than that of fertile eggs laid by nominally unrelated pairs, 67.1 percent and 57.5 percent respectively. At least 15 eggs laid at the Government Aviaries have lacked yolks, all but four of them laid by two females.

Infertile eggs have been found in the wild. Two out of ten Pink Pigeon eggs collected for the captive breeding programme proved to be infertile. One pair of pigeons released at Pamplemousses laid two clutches of infertile eggs.

Embryonic mortality

In the two captive populations, embryonic mortality accounts for the failure of

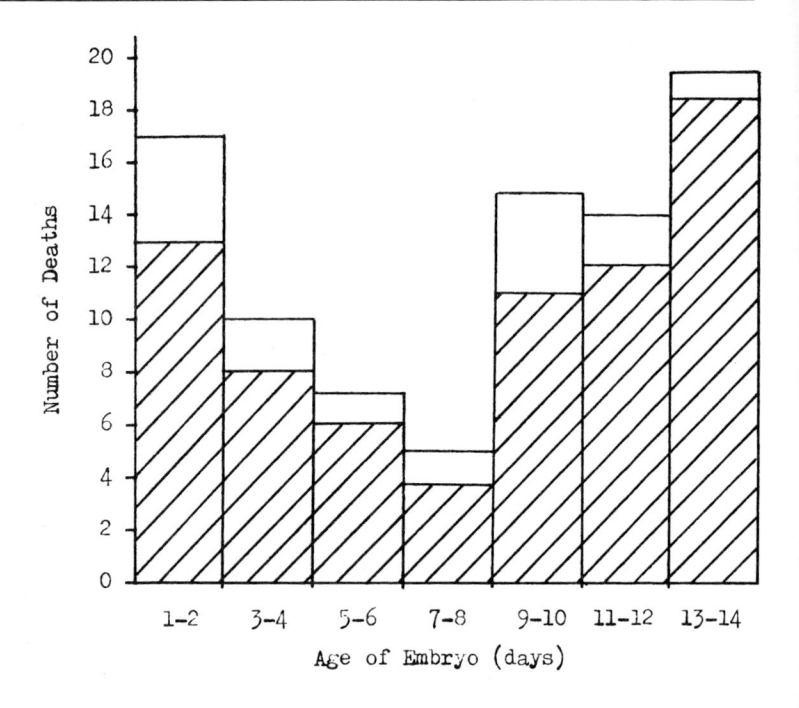

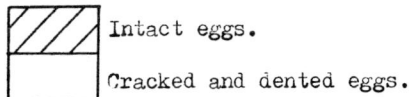

[Figure: bar chart showing Number of Deaths vs Age of Embryo (days), with bins 1-2, 3-4, 5-6, 7-8, 9-10, 11-12, 13-14. Hatched portions represent Intact eggs; unhatched portions represent Cracked and dented eggs.]

Figure 6: Age distribution of 87 embryo deaths in the captive Pink Pigeon population at the Government Aviaries.

a third of all fertile eggs. The age distribution of 87 embryo deaths at the Government Aviaries is shown in *Figure 6*. There are two peaks, one early and one late in incubation, a pattern similar to that described for the Domestic Pigeon (Riddle 1930) and the Domestic Chicken (*Gallus gallus*) (Gordon 1977). At the Government Aviaries, 39 percent of Pink Pigeon deaths occurred during the first six days and 56 percent during the last six days of the 14-day incubation period. Eighteen percent of embryonic deaths occurred during hatching, compared with 14 percent at the JWPT (Rankine 1983).

Eggs with minor cracks, dents or holes when removed from the parental nest have been repaired with nail-varnish. Over 70 percent of the fertile eggs among them died before hatching, probably from either bacterial infection or faulty water balance. No gross abnormalities have been detected when unhatched eggs have been opened to age the dead embryo, though detailed examination may reveal minor defects. The incidence of infectious disease in the egg is not known, while desertion has caused the loss of fewer than five eggs at the Government Aviaries.

Squab mortality
In the captive populations, 46.9 percent of Pink Pigeons hatched have died

before the age of 30 days. At the Government Aviaries, two-thirds (68.5 percent) of the squab deaths occurred within four days of hatching and 83.8 percent by the tenth day. A similar pattern of mortality is evident in the JWPT data (*Figure 7*).

Possible causes of the deaths of 156 Pink Pigeon squabs are listed in *Table 7*. In over a third of cases, the cause of death has not been identified. Faulty management techniques and accidents accounted for about a quarter of the deaths, while developmental problems and poor or incompetent parental care contributed about 17 percent and 12 percent respectively. Infectious disease apparently played a comparatively minor role although it must be stressed that full microbiological investigations were not made. The early peaks in mortality shown in *Figure 7* are largely accounted for by the deaths with no apparent cause, combined with the deaths of squabs that were weak at hatching and those poorly synchronized to their foster-parents on Mauritius, and with the deaths due to chilling at JWPT.

The deaths of squabs that were very weak at hatching, in some cases requiring to be helped from the shell, and which never improved, have been tentatively attributed to faulty development in *Table 7*, even though the possibly diverse causes of 'weakness' have not been identified. Of the other developmental defects which have proved fatal to squabs, the most common has been incomplete absorption of the yolk-sac. The exposed yolk-sac is vulnerable to damage and infection.

The other developmental defects are discussed below.

Deaths during foster- and hand-rearing

Sixteen Pink Pigeon squabs have died at the Government Aviaries because they were poorly synchronized with their foster parents' incubation cycle, and were either fed crop-milk adulterated with seeds or just seeds and water. If this happens, the squabs may suffer from intestinal blockage or peritonitis and will die if not treated promptly (Jones *et al*. 1983).

The foster doves cease feeding the young Pink Pigeon at about two and a half to three weeks if they fail to solicit food vigorously. Occasionally squabs will not have started feeding themselves by this stage and would starve if not hand-reared. Hand-rearing of these older squabs has ended in the deaths of six of them following crop rupture. Squabs used to be fed by syringing food directly into the crop via a plastic tube placed down the oesophagus (Jones *et al*. 1983), but this occasionally led to damage to the crop lining if the bird struggled or was inadvertently handled too roughly. This source of mortality has now been eliminated by the adoption of a shorter feeding tube.

INBREEDING DEPRESSION

The captive Pink Pigeons are descended from eleven birds from the wild. At no time since the first one was caught in 1976 has the wild population been estimated to comprise more than 30 birds (Jones 1987) and it is probable that some of the founder stock were related. The captive populations could therefore include many more inbred birds than those known. (For the calculation of kinship and inbreeding coefficients used in this paper, it has had to be assumed that no wild-bred Pink Pigeon in captivity was related to another.)

Early in the captive breeding programme, a large proportion of Pink Pigeons at the Government Aviaries were the young of a particularly productive pair.

Death attributed to:
- unknown / unidentified
- very weak at hatching
- poorly synchronised
- chilling
- other

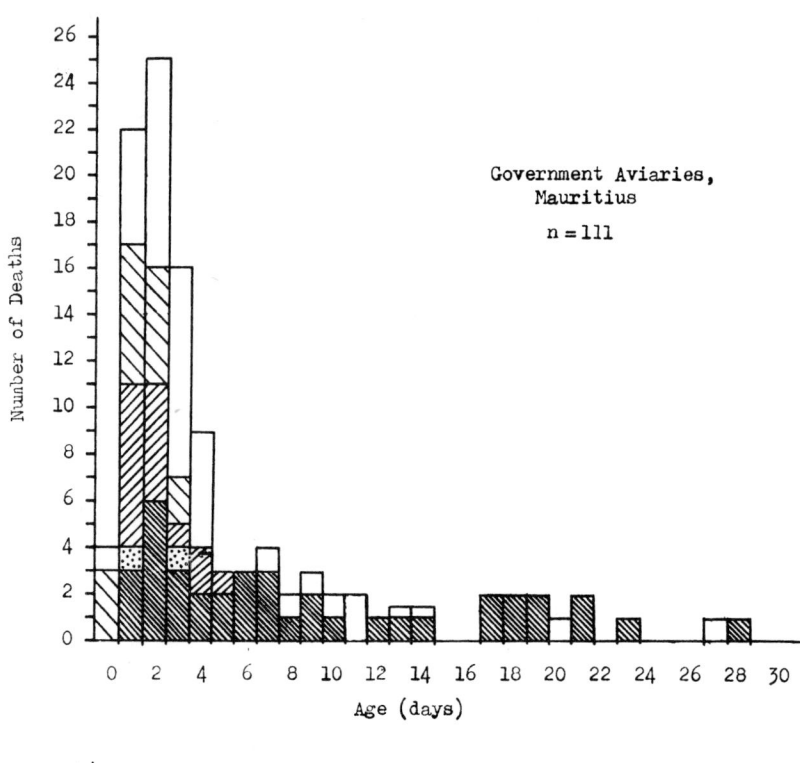

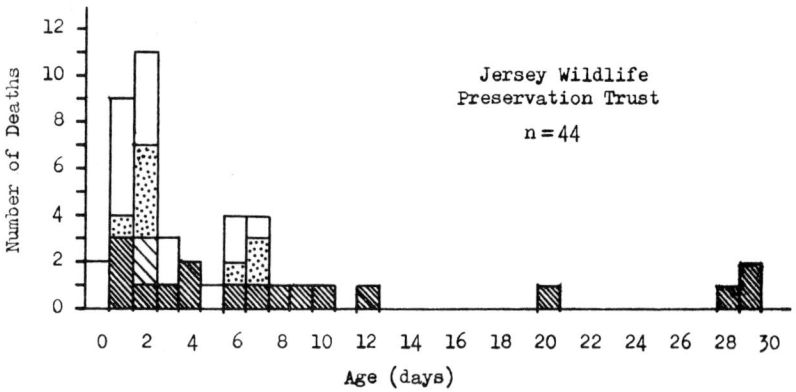

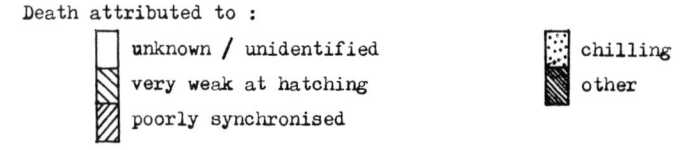

Figure 7: Age distribution of Pink Pigeon squab deaths at the Government Aviaries and at the Jersey Wildlife Preservation Trust.

Table 7: Causes of Pink Pigeon squab mortality at the Government Aviaries and the JWPT.

Proximate or Contributory Causes	Government Aviaries	JWPT	Total No.	%
Unknown/Unidentified	38	17	55	35.3
Management and accidents	39	3	42	26.9
Poorly synchronized with foster-parents	16	0		
Incorrect diet when hand-reared	11	1		
Ruptured crop	6	0		
Accident (fracture, entangled foot, etc.)	3	2		
Internal haemorrhage	3	0		
Developmental problems	19	7	26	16.7
Very weak at hatching	16	2		
Incomplete yolk-sac absorption	1	4		
'Spontaneous' fractures	1	0		
Ataxia	1	0		
Undersized and underdeveloped	0	1		
Incompetent parental behaviour	7	11	18	11.6
Fell from nest	4	1		
Chilling	2	8		
Crushed by (foster-)parent	1	1		
Injured by father	0	1		
Infectious diseases	5	6	11	7.1
Congested lungs/pneumonia	0	2		
Coliform infection	0	2		
Cloacitis	2	0		
? Coccidiosis	1	0		
Caseous lesions in intestines and lungs	1	0		
Corynebacterium infection	0	1		
Trichomoniasis	0	1		
Severe eye infection	1	0		
Predation, etc.	4	0	4	2.6
Black Rat (*Rattus rattus*)	1	0		
Larvae of Tropical Nest Fly (*Passeromyia heterochaeta*)	3	0		
TOTAL	112	44	156	

As a result, a number of pairs of siblings were allowed to breed. In *Table 8* and *Figure 8*, the fate of eggs from sib matings or their equivalent (kinship coefficient 0.25) is compared with that of eggs laid by pairs not known to be related. Eggs from pairs including a bird known to be inbred have been excluded. The fertility of eggs from related pairs was found to be higher than that of eggs from nominally unrelated pairs, though the difference is not significant at the 5 percent level. In contrast, the proportions of fertile, unbroken eggs that hatch, squabs that fledge, and fledglings that survive for one year, are all significantly lower for the inbred eggs. These results are not unexpected as the deleterious effects of inbreeding on normally outbreeding populations are now well documented (e.g. Wright 1977; Senner 1980). The possible presence of related birds in the founder stock and the unrecorded inbreeding which would have resulted could account for the relatively poor breeding results shown by the nominally unrelated pairs.

Table 8: The effect of inbreeding on the breeding success of the Pink Pigeons at the Government Aviaries.

	Nominally unrelated pairs		Sib matings or equivalent				
	No.	%	No.	%	n	χ^2	P
No. of pairs	23		17				
No. of eggs	592		191				
No. (%) smashed	110	18.6	41	21.5	783	0.598	n.s.
No. (%) fertile	263/457	57.5	96/143	67.1	600	3.773	n.s.
Est. no. of fertile, unsmashed eggs	277		101				
No. (%) hatched	194	70.0	58	57.4	378	4.744	<0.05
No. (%) fledged	117	60.3	24	41.4	252	5.747	<0.05
No. (%) to one year	88	75.2	11	45.8	141	6.875	<0.01

DISCUSSION

In the two major captive populations of Pink Pigeons, mortality has followed a pattern common to many species of bird, both wild (free-living) and captive (e.g. Lack 1954; Hillgarth & Kear 1981). However, the percentage of individuals dying at each stage of the breeding cycle has been higher than that found in most other studies.

A number of conditions affecting Pink Pigeons have been recognized. In some cases their probable causes can be inferred due to their similarity to known conditions in Domestic Pigeons or other well studied species. A few of those exhibited by Pink Pigeons appear to be solely genetic in origin, for example 'cleft tail feathers'; others such as 'clubbed down' and 'crooked toe deformity', are primarily thought to be the result of dietary deficiencies or poor management, although their individual expression may be influenced by the genetic background of the individual.

Nutritional deficiencies

Several nutritional problems have been diagnosed in the Pink Pigeons on Mauritius, and two of the most important of these have been pantothenic acid and vitamin A deficiencies. A deficiency of vitamin A may have been the cause of nervous problems in several birds. In chickens, vitamin A deficiency has been reported as causing degenerative changes in both the central and peripheral nervous systems resulting in ataxia and incoordination (Siegmund 1979; Gordon 1977). Although not necessarily fatal, a deficiency of vitamin A reduces the bird's viability and may leave it more susceptible to infections.

Vitamin A deficiencies have been largely avoided in recent years on Mauritius because the pigeons are now provided with maize on a regular basis. The original diet would in theory have met the vitamin A requirements of Domestic Pigeons (Levi 1978), and the foster Barbary Doves provided with the same diet as the Pink Pigeon have never shown signs of deficiency. It is therefore possible that both Domestic Pigeons and Barbary Doves, which usually feed on seeds low in vitamin A, are adapted to the low levels of this vitamin. Consequently they are likely to be very efficient at absorbing it whereas the Pink Pigeons which eat a wider range of foodstuffs, many of which are very high in vitamin A, do not have to have such efficient rates of absorption or metabolism.

The diet provided for the Pink Pigeons at the Government Aviaries may be

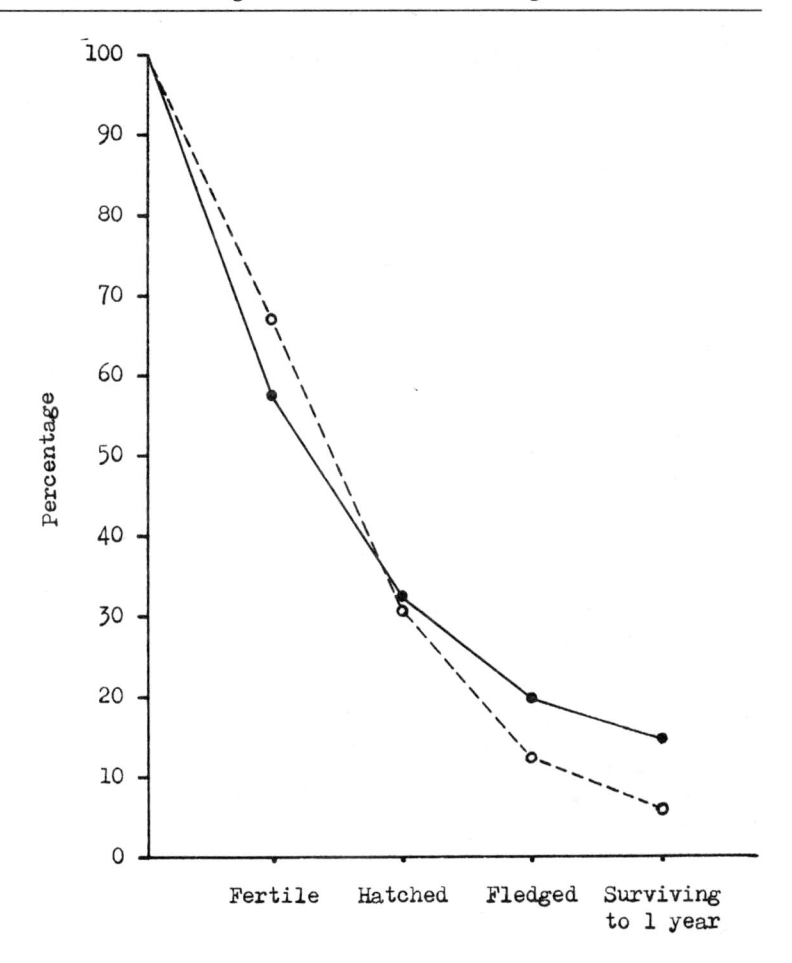

●——● Nominally unrelated pairs.

○——○ Sib matings or their equivalent.

Figure 8: The breeding success of 23 nominally unrelated pairs of Pink Pigeons and 17 pairs of siblings or their equivalent (kinship coefficient = 0.25).

too high in protein. This is suggested by the incidence of kidney lesions, including interstitial nephritis, recorded post mortem (Cooper *et al.* 1987) and the one case of articular gout. The occurrence of 'splayed legs' and 'slipped wing' may also be due to the same dietary imbalance, though these conditions have alternatively been attributed to calcium and phosphorus deficiencies (Kear 1973, 1978).

Although dietary deficiencies might have been having a general effect depressing the viability of the pigeons, this does not appear to be the case. Conditions caused by deficiencies, for example of vitamin A, have developed, but improving the diet has not led to a marked improvement in the breeding results, even though the incidence of these conditions has dropped significantly. There has also been great variation in fertility between pairs and in mortality between their offspring, even though all birds have been provided with the same diet.

Developmental conditions

A common skeletal deformity that has affected the Pink Pigeons has been 'inclined feet'—a condition that may be homologous to club foot. Jones *et al.* (1983) suggested that the condition was the result of shortened flexor tendons, because the foot is twisted even further inwards if an attempt is made to straighten the leg. Cooper *et al.* (1987) and Flach (1984) have described the condition post mortem. The main deformity identified was a rotation of the distal end of the tarsometatarsus causing an associated malpositioning of the tendons. Cooper *et al.* (1987) could find no evidence of bone disease in radiographs, but could not exclude the possibility that skeletal lesions at an early age played a part. Jones *et al.* (1983) speculated that 'inclined foot' was of genetic origin, but examination of the family tree of the captive Pink Pigeon population has failed to support this. 'Curled toe paralysis', a condition affecting poultry and other bird species, has similarities to 'inclined feet'. It is caused by riboflavin deficiency and is associated with enlargement of the sheaths of the sciatic and brachial nerves (Scott *et al.* 1982). The nerves of Pink Pigeons with 'inclined feet' have not yet been examined to establish the homology of this condition. However, none of the offspring of the pair which produced young with 'clubbed down' has developed 'inclined feet'.

The most common skeletal deformity is a bent or wavy sternum. The condition is well known in a range of bird species including the Domestic Pigeon. Levi (1977) considered that the deformity was the result of an unsuitable nest-substrate and an inadequate diet. He also noted that some breeds are more susceptible to the condition than others, suggesting that genetic factors are involved in its aetiology.

'Adrenal stress'

Subordinate birds in pairs or groups often feed less or stop feeding completely and die from inanition or secondary conditions. Murton *et al.* (1971) described an apparently similar cause of mortality in wild Wood Pigeons (*Columba palumbus*), in which subordinate birds lost weight and died from inanition and adrenal stress. Examination post mortem revealed hyperplasia of the cortical cells of the adrenal glands. The adrenal glands of the Pink Pigeons that died in the circumstances described above have not yet been examined in detail, so the possible homology of these conditions cannot be confirmed.

Breeding success

Jenkins *et al.* (this volume) attribute the high rates of infertility and mortality at all stages in the wild population of Hawaiian Crows (*Corvus hawaiiensis*) to exotic diseases, in particular to avian malaria and avian pox. There is, however, no evidence to date that infectious disease is a major factor reducing the breeding success of the Pink Pigeons.

In *Tables 5* and *9*, the breeding success of the wild population of Pink Pigeons is compared with that of some other pigeon and dove species. In the studies used for comparison, the percentage of eggs producing fledglings ranges from almost 70 percent in the Collared Dove (*Streptopelia decaocto*) to less than 10 percent in the Pink Pigeon. At less than 10 percent, the proportion of Pink

Table 9: Nesting success of wild Pink Pigeons compared with that of some other pigeon and dove species.

Species	No. of nests	No. of young fledged	% nests fledging young	Young fledging per nest	Young per successful nest
Pink Pigeon					
Columba (Nesoenas) mayeri	14	1	7.1	0.07	1.0
—Mauritius	c.35	0	0	0	0
	48	4	≤8.3	0.08	1.0(?)
	68	≤8	?	≤0.12	?
Stock Dove *C.oenas*	399	c.519	c.73	1.3	1.78
—East Germany					
Laughing Dove *Streptopelia*					
senegalensis—South Africa	619	c.433	?	0.7	?
—Botswana	672	c.591	?	0.88	?
Mourning Dove *Zenaida*					
macroura—USA	249	c.213	52.2	0.86	1.64
—USA	204	c.274	69.7	1.34	1.93
Ruddy Ground Dove	21	8	23.8	0.38	1.60
Columbina talpacoti—Costa Rica					
Cold-billed Ground Dove	283	(263)	56.5	c.0.93	c.1.64
C.cruziana—Ecuador					

Notes: Data for the Pink Pigeon are from McKelvey (1976, 1977), Temple (1978) and Jones (1987). Data for the other species are from Cramp (1985) and Ricklefs (1969) who refer to various original sources.

Pigeon nests fledging young is also low. With the exception of the Ruddy Ground Dove (*Columbia talpacoti*), the other species for which figures are available fledge young from over 50 percent of their nests. Predation is a major cause of nest failure in some of the other studies, but in no case where detailed figures are provided does it approach the level suffered by the Pink Pigeons. Pink Pigeons might be expected to be especially vulnerable to mammalian predators having evolved on an island with none, even though they do have a nest distraction display (McKelvey 1976; Jones 1987).

Observations and some experimental evidence support the suggestion that the introduced Long-tailed Macaque (*Macaca fascicularis*) is the main nest-predator (McKelvey 1976, 1977; Jones 1987). McKelvey, for example, reported the loss of 40 out of 48 nests to macaques during 1976. Although there is no direct evidence, Ship Rats (*Rattus rattus*) probably destroy some clutches as well. They are known nest-predators (Atkinson 1978) and have been recorded taking the eggs of other Mauritian bird species (Jones 1987). The only extant native nest-predator is the Mauritian Cuckoo-shrike (*Coracina typica*), which was reported to have taken four out of 48 clutches of Pink Pigeon eggs in 1976 (McKelvey 1977).

The incidence of infertile eggs has been greater than might be expected and occurs about three times more frequently than in Domestic Pigeons (*Table 4*). The difference may be even greater since Levi (1977) considered that only 3 percent to 5 percent of Domestic Pigeon eggs were infertile and that the numbers reported were too high because they included eggs which failed due to early embryonic death.

The prevalence of embryonic death in Pink Pigeons is also exceptionally high compared with that recorded in Domestic Pigeons, in which less than 5 percent of fertile eggs died (Levi 1977). Although these data came from squab breeding

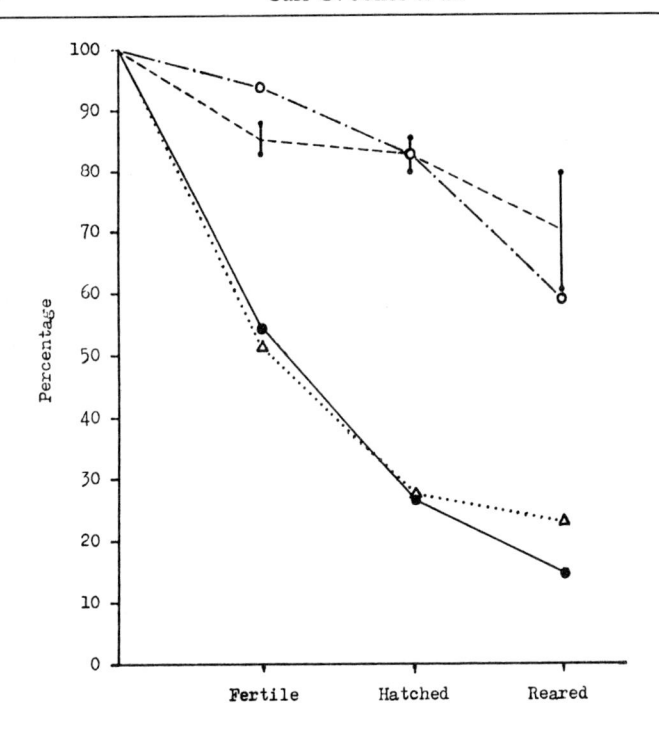

●——● Pink Pigeon. Data from populations at the Government Aviaries and JWPT. 'Reared' refers to birds reaching an age of 30 days.

|---| Domestic Pigeon. Ranges cover results from four years of the New Jersey Squab Breeding Contest and one year at the Chaffey Squab Breeding Experimental Station Contest. 'Reared' refers to marketable birds (25 - 35 days old) (reviewed in Levi 1978).

o—·—o Feral Pigeon. Data excluding predated nests adapted from Murton & Clarke 1968. 'Reared' refers to birds fledged.

△········△ Hawaiian Goose. Data from captive population at the Wildfowl Trust, 1962 - 1972 (Kear & Berger 1980).

Figure 9: Breeding success of the Pink Pigeon compared with that of Domestic and Feral Pigeons (*Columba livia*) and Hawaiian Geese (*Branta sandvicensis*).

contests and so might be expected to be inflated, this does not seem to be the case. Comparable figures were obtained by excluding the figures for predated nests from data on Feral Pigeons (also *C. livia*) in Murton & Clarke (1968) (*Figure 9*). The Pink Pigeon results are similar to those recorded for an inbred population of another endangered island species in captivity, the Hawaiian Goose (*Branta sandvicensis*) at The Wildfowl Trust, England (Kear & Berger 1980).

A deficiency of either vitamin A or riboflavin, both of which have been suspected in squabs at the Government Aviaries, reduces the hatchability of chickens' eggs (Scott *et al.* 1982) and may account for some Pink Pigeon embryo mortality.

The prevalence of squab mortality is far higher than that found in the Domestic

Pigeon squab breeding contests which Levi (1978) reports as ranging from 6.9 percent to 24.3 percent *(Table 4)*.

Squabs less than five days old, which are not being fed properly by their foster-parents, have proved difficult to rear by hand. Many of the early attempts ended in failure, probably because the high carbohydrate content of the artificial diets used reversed the osmotic gradient in the gut causing dehydration (Jones *et al.* 1983). Mammalian milk compares well with crop milk as a source of protein, fatty acids and some vitamins, but it contains lactose. Pigeons do not produce lactase and mammalian milk should therefore not be fed to squabs (*contra* Jones *et al.* 1983), since it may ferment in the gut. A shortage of manganese, which birds require in greater quantities than mammals, may be another cause of failure to hand-rear young squabs (Jones *et al.* 1983).

Inbreeding depression

If an ultimate cause of the poor breeding results is to be identified, inbreeding depression is the most likely candidate. The Pink Pigeons have exhibited many of the effects of inbreeding depression described for other species, such as poor parental behaviour, decreased fertility, low hatchability of fertile eggs, poor survival of young, and increased susceptibility to a wide range of apparently unrelated diseases, both infectious and non-infectious (Soulé 1980; Senner 1980; Ralls *et al.* 1980). These deleterious effects are, however, not confined to those Pink Pigeons known to be inbred. It is therefore probable that some, if not all, of the pigeons taken from the wild were related. As the wild population is small and has recently declined in numbers, it may also be suffering from the effects of inbreeding, though these would be masked to a large extent by the high level of nest predation.

In *Figure 9*, the breeding success of the Pink Pigeons at the Government Aviaries and the JWPT is compared with that of the Hawaiian Geese at The Wildfowl Trust between 1952 and 1972. In the first ten years, the latter population was highly inbred, all birds being descended from just three founder birds. However, over the next five years four males from Hawaii were introduced (Kear & Berger 1980). For the first ten years breeding success was worse than that of the Pink Pigeons, but with the arrival of the new males, it improved significantly. It is therefore only by coincidence that the composite results match the breeding success of the Pink Pigeon so closely. However, the fact that the breeding success of the Pink Pigeons has been depressed in a similar pattern to that shown by a population known to be highly inbred supports the hypothesis that unrecorded inbreeding is reducing the viability of the captive birds.

In an investigation of the breeding records of a herd of captive Dorcas Gazelles (*Gazella dorcas*), Ralls *et al.* (1980) found that inbred calves had died due to premature birth, inanition and a variety of miscellaneous medical problems and infections, none of which had caused the death of non-inbred calves. The situation is not so clear cut in Pink Pigeons. The only causes of death to which inbred squabs succumbed in significantly higher numbers than expected were 'weakness' and being fed on an unsuitable artificial diet. These are related since in many cases weak squabs needed to be hand-fed. There is no obvious correlation between inbreeding and particular causes of death of fledged Pink Pigeons.

ACKNOWLEDGEMENTS

Carl Jones is sponsored by the Jersey Wildlife Preservation Trust/Wildlife

Preservation Trust International and manages their projects on Mauritius. David Todd was sponsored between 1984 and 1988 by the Jersey Wildlife Preservation Trust and Wildlife Preservation Trust Canada to work on Pink Pigeons. Yousoof Mungroo is Scientific Officer in the Conservation Unit of the Ministry of Agriculture. We are all most grateful to our respective organizations for their help and encouragement.

The Government Aviaries at Black River are run by the Department of Forestry, and we are grateful to Mr. Wahab Owadally, Conservator of Forests, for all his help and support. The Pink Pigeon captive breeding programme on Mauritius is now financed by the Government of Mauritius and the Jersey Wildlife Preservation Trust/Wildlife Preservation Trust. The New York Zoological Society, the International Council for Bird Preservation, and both International World Wildlife Fund and the United States national section have given their support in the past.

J. E. Cooper at the Royal College of Surgeons of England has been the veterinary advisor to the project since its inception and we are grateful to him for his advice and for allowing us to make use of his pathological results.

Dr Christine Halais read a draft of this paper and her comments have been most valuable. We would also like to thank an anonymous reviewer for some helpful advice.

REFERENCES

ARNALL, L. & KEYMER, I. F. 1975. *Bird Diseases*. Baillière Tindall, London.

ATKINSON, I. A. E. 1978. Evidence of effects of rodents on the vertebrate wildlife of New Zealand islands. *In*: Dingwall, P. R., Atkinson, I. A. E. & Hay, C. *The ecology and control of rodents in New Zealand nature reserves*. Dept. Lands & Survey, Info. Series 4, Wellington.

COOPER, J. E., NEEDHAM, J. R., APPLEBEE, K. & JONES, C. G. 1987. Clinical and pathological studies on the Mauritian Pink Pigeon (*Columba mayeri*). *Ibis* **130**: 57–64.

CRAMP, S. (ed.) 1985. *Birds of the Western Palaearctic*. Vol. IV.—*Terns to Woodpeckers*. Oxford Univ. Press.

FLACH, E. J. 1984. *Observations, clinical examinations and post-mortem examinations on two Mayer's Pink Pigeons, Nesoenas mayeri, with locomotor disorders*. Report of Summer School Project, Jersey Wildlife Preservation Trust.

GORDON, R. F. 1977. *Poultry Diseases*. Baillière Tindall, London.

HILLGARTH, N. & KEAR, J. 1981. Diseases of perching ducks in captivity. *Wildfowl* **32**: 156–63.

JENKINS, C. D., TEMPLE, S. A., VAN RIPER C. & HANSEN, W. R. (this volume) Disease-related aspects of conserving the endangered Hawaiian Crow.

JONES, C. G. 1987. The larger land-birds of Mauritius. *In*: Diamond, A. W. (ed.). *Studies on Mascarene Island birds*. Cambridge Univ. Press, Cambridge.

JONES, C. G., JEGGO, D. F. & HARTLEY, J. 1983. The maintenance and captive breeding of the Pink Pigeon *(Nesoenas mayeri)*. *Dodo, J. Jersey Wildl. Preserv. Trust* **20**: 16–26.

KEAR, J. 1973. Notes on the nutrition of young waterfowl, with special reference to slipped-wing. *Int. Zoo. Ybk.* **13**: 97–100.

KEAR, J. 1978. Feeding and nutrition. *In*: Fowler, M. E. (ed.). *Zoo and Wild Animal Medicine* W.B. Saunders, Philadelphia.

KEAR, J. & BERGER, A. J. 1980. *The Hawaiian Goose—an Experiment in Conservation*. T. & A. D. Poyser, Calton.

KREEGER, T. J. & WALSER, M. M. 1984. Carpometacarpal deformity in Giant Canada Geese (*Branta canadensis maxima* Delacour). *J. Wildl. Dis.* **20** (3): 245–8.

LACK, D. 1954. *The Natural Regulation of Animal Numbers*. Oxford University Press, Oxford.

LEVI, W. M. 1977. *The pigeon*. Levi Publishing Co., Sumter, S. C.

MCKELVEY, S. D. 1976. A preliminary study of the Mauritian Pink Pigeon (*Nesoenas mayeri*). *Mauritius Inst. Bull.* **8** (2): 145–75.

MCKELVEY, S. D. 1977. Some observations on the Mauritian Pink Pigeon. *Birds Internat.* **2**: 36–8.

MURTON, R. K. & CLARKE, S. P. 1968. Breeding biology of Rock Doves. *Br. Birds* **61**: 429–48.

MURTON, R. K., ISAACSON, A. J. & WESTWOOD, N. J. 1971. The significance of gregarious feeding behaviour and adrenal stress in a population of Wood-pigeons *Columba palumbus*. *J. Zool.* **165**: 53–84.

PEIRCE, M. A. 1984. Haematozoa of African birds: some miscellaneous findings. *Afr. J. Ecol.* **22**: 149–52.

PEIRCE, M. A., CHEKE, A. S. & CHEKE, R. A. 1977. A survey of blood parasites of birds in the Mascarene Islands, Indian Ocean. *Ibis* **119**: 451–61.

RALLS, K., BRUGGER, K. & GLICK, A. 1980. Deleterious effects of inbreeding in a herd of captive Dorcas Gazelle *Gazella dorcas*. *Int. Zoo Ybk.* **20**: 137–46.

RANKINE, J. 1983. *Analysis of breeding records of the Pink Pigeon* (Nesoenas mayeri) *at the JWPT and Black River, Mauritius*. Unpublished report to JWPT.

RICKLEFS, R. E. 1969. An analysis of nesting mortality in birds. *Smithsonian Contributions to Zoology*, no. 9. Washington DC.

RIDDLE, O. 1930. Studies on the physiology of reproduction in birds. XXVII—The age distribution of mortality in bird embryos and its probable significance. *Amer. J. Physiol.* **94**: 535–47.

SCOTT, M. L., NESHEIM, M. C. & YOUNG, R. J. 1982. *Nutrition of the Chicken*. M. L. Scott & Associates, Ithaca, N.Y.

SENNER, J. W. 1980. Inbreeding depression and the survival of zoo populations. *In*: Soulé, M. E. & Wilcox, B. A., (eds). *Conservation Biology: an Evolutionary-ecological Perspective*. Sinauer Associates, Sunderland, Mass.

SIEGMUND, H. (ed.) 1979. *The Merck Veterinary Manual*. N. J. Merck & Co., Rahway.

SNYDER, B., THILSTEAD, J., BURGESS, B. & RICHARD, M. 1985. Pigeon herpesvirus mortalities in foster reared Mauritius Pink Pigeons. *Abstracts and Papers—1985 Annual Meeting, American Association of Zoo Veterinarians*, Arizona.

SOULÉ, M. E. 1980. Thresholds for survival: maintaining fitness and evolutionary potential. *In*: Soulé, M. E. & Wilcox, B. A. (eds). *Conservation Biology: an Evolutionary-ecological Perspective*. Sinauer Associates, Sunderland, Mass.

TEMPLE, S. A. 1978. *The life histories and ecology of the indigenous landbirds of Mauritius*. Unpubl. manuscript.

TODD, D. M. 1984. The release of Pink Pigeons *Columba* (*Nesoenas*) *mayeri* at Pamplemousses, Mauritius. *Dodo, J. Jersey Wildl. Preserv. Trust* **21**: 43–57.

WRIGHT, S. 1977. *Evolution and Genetics of Populations*. Vol. III—*Experimental Results and Evolutionary Deductions*. Univ. of Chicago Press, Chicago.

THE IMPACT OF EASTERN EQUINE ENCEPHALITIS VIRUS ON EFFORTS TO RECOVER THE ENDANGERED WHOOPING CRANE

JAMES W. CARPENTER,[1] GARY G. CLARK[2] & DOUGLAS M. WATTS[2]

1 *Endangered Species Research Branch, Patuxent Wildlife Research Center, U.S. Fish and Wildlife Service, Laurel, Maryland 20708, USA.*
2 *Department of Arboviral Entomology, U.S. Army Medical Research Institute of Infectious Diseases, Fort Detrick, Frederick, Maryland 21701, USA.*

ABSTRACT

The Whooping Crane (*Grus americana*), although never abundant in North America, became endangered primarily because of habitat modification and destruction. To help recovery, a captive propagation and reintroduction programme was initiated at the Patuxent Wildlife Research Center (PWRC) in 1966. However, in 1984, 7 of 39 Whooping Cranes at PWRC died from infection by eastern equine encephalitis (EEE) virus, an arbovirus that infects a wide variety of indigenous bird species, although mortality is generally restricted to introduced birds. Following identification of the aetiological agent, surveillance and control measures were implemented, including serological monitoring of both wild and captive birds for EEE viral antibody and assay of locally-trapped mosquitoes for virus. In addition, an inactivated EEE virus vaccine developed for use in humans was evaluated in captive Whooping Cranes. Results so far suggest that the vaccine will afford protection to susceptible birds.

As part of the effort to restore Whooping Crane populations in the wild, three geographically isolated areas in the eastern USA are being considered as possible reintroduction sites. Since EEE viral transmission occurs annually in parts of the eastern USA, it will be important to survey for EEE virus and its vectors before selecting the release sites.

Although the die-off of Whooping Cranes due to the EEE virus was a setback for the captive breeding programme, we now know that this disease must be considered in establishing wild crane populations. However, through monitoring and research efforts, it appears that the adverse effects of EEE virus on Whooping Crane recovery can be minimized.

INTRODUCTION

Prior to European colonization of North America, the breeding range of the Whooping Crane (*Grus americana*) extended from Illinois northwestward through Iowa, Minnesota, North Dakota, Manitoba, Saskatchewan and Alberta (U.S. Fish and Wildlife Service 1986). A local, disjunct breeding population, believed to have been nonmigratory, also occurred in Louisiana. By the 1890s, the Whooping Crane no longer bred in the north-central United States. The only remaining wild population wintered each year in Texas, then migrated to an unknown breeding ground. After the last known nesting record in Canada in 1922, three decades elapsed until the breeding site of the remnant population was discovered in 1954 in the Northwest Territories.

The Whooping Crane is included in the United States *'List of Endangered and Threatened Wildlife and Plants'* (Title 50, Code of Federal Regulations, Part 17), implying that the species is in imminent danger of extinction unless management is successful in assuring its preservation. Two primary factors led to the decline of the Whooping Crane: 1) man's conversion of prairie potholes and surrounding areas to agriculture made nearly all of the habitat in its original range unsuitable for the species, and 2) hunting and specimen collecting directly reduced Whooping Crane numbers (Allen 1952).

The Whooping Crane also has delayed sexual maturity (breeding at approximately five to six years) and a small clutch size (normally two eggs) which compound the adverse impacts of human settlement on its population numbers. In addition, the northern breeding grounds are ice-free for only four months each year (U.S. Fish and Wildlife Service 1986). During the breeding season, therefore, adverse weather and limitations on food supply may disrupt breeding attempts, and seldom is there enough time for cranes to lay a second clutch and fledge young before cold weather sets in again.

Cooperative management activities by the United States and Canada, including habitat protection, public education, legislation, law enforcement, captive propagation, and intensive research and management, have resulted in a gradual increase in Whooping Crane numbers from a low of 21 birds in 1941 to approximately 165, including both wild (free-living) and captive populations, in early 1986. Contributing to this increase has been the attempt to establish a second Whooping Crane population in Idaho. To establish this population, Whooping Crane eggs have, since 1975, been placed in Sandhill Crane (*Grus canadensis*) nests and reared by foster parents at Grays Lake National Wildlife Refuge.

This second Whooping Crane population now numbers approximately 30 individuals which summer in Idaho and surrounding states and winter primarily in New Mexico. At present, Florida, Georgia and Michigan are being evaluated as sites for a third Whooping Crane population. Thus, establishment of additional, self-sustaining, geographically isolated Whooping Crane populations is intended to increase the prospects for survival (Erickson & Derrickson 1981).

The Endangered Species Research Program was established at the Patuxent Wildlife Research Center (PWRC) in 1965 by the U.S. Fish and Wildlife Service. The programme was designed to give special attention to severely threatened or declining species whose future could not be assured by existing protection and management methods (Erickson 1968). The objectives of this research programme were two-fold: (1) to identify and evaluate environmental and biological limiting factors through field and laboratory investigations; and (2) to augment or establish wild populations through captive propagation. The Whooping Crane has received the most public and scientific attention of the eight species at PWRC that have been successfully propagated and reintroduced to the wild.

CLINICAL AND PATHOLOGICAL FEATURES

Between September and November, 1984, 7 of 39 Whooping Cranes at PWRC died. Four birds were found dead without any clinical signs, and three showed signs of lethargy, ataxia, and neck and leg paresis prior to death. Medical treatment that was provided to the three clinically ill cranes included hospitalization and supportive therapy. Complete blood counts, serum chemistries, and faecal examinations were also performed. In contrast, no clinical signs or mortality were observed in the 248 Sandhill Cranes that were located in pens interspersed among the Whooping Crane pens (Dein *et al.* 1986; Carpenter *et al.* 1987).

Complete post-mortem examinations were performed on all seven birds. The only significant gross lesions were an accumulation of clear yellow fluid in the anterior (cranial) abdominal air sacs of three birds, and enlarged livers in four others. Histopathological examination revealed a diffuse inflammatory response with necrosis throughout many organs with no inclusion bodies. Bacterial and chlamydial cultures produced no significant growth. Tissue and feed samples were negative for selected heavy metals, pesticides, and biotoxins. However, a suspected viral agent from post-mortem samples including liver, lung, spleen and kidneys was identified as a member of the family Togaviridae by electron-microscopic examination and as EEE virus by serological assays (Dein *et al.* 1986; Carpenter *et al.* 1987). Among the surviving Whooping Cranes, 14 (44 percent) of 32, as well as 13 (34 percent) of 38 Sandhill Cranes, were positive for neutralizing antibody to EEE virus.

OTHER INVESTIGATIONS

Following identification of the aetiological agent, ground and air reconnaissance was conducted at PWRC and adjacent areas to determine the presence and distribution of potential arthropod vectors. Surveillance and control measures were directed toward *Culiseta melanura* (Diptera) and other possible vectors of EEE virus, and included serological monitoring of both wild and captive birds for EEE viral antibody. Mosquitoes were collected, identified, and assayed for viral antigen. Seronegative Bobwhite Quail (*Colinus virginianus*) and Sandhill Cranes were bled biweekly and serum was assayed for neutralizing antibody to EEE virus. Research to assess the safety and efficacy of an inactivated human EEE virus vaccine for captive Whooping Cranes was also initiated (Carpenter *et al.* 1987; Dein *et al.* 1986; Clark *et al.* 1987).

RESULTS

The mosquitoes sampled were all negative for virus and none of the birds examined showed any titre to EEE virus. Following intramuscular administration and two booster doses of vaccine, Whooping Cranes developed moderately high neutralizing antibody titres (1:80–1:320) to EEE virus.

DISCUSSION

EEE virus causes sporadic disease outbreaks in humans and in certain avian and mammalian species. The virus is transmitted to birds primarily by *Culiseta melanura* and to a lesser degree by *Coquillettidia perturbans*—both mosquitoes found in freshwater swamp habitats (Williams *et al.* 1972). Numerous species of wild bird are the principal hosts for amplifying the EEE virus (Kissling et al. 1954; Stamm 1963). An EEE viraemia, sufficient to infect susceptible female mosquitoes, is present for three to five days, beginning two to three days after the birds have been infected. Passerine birds, particularly nestlings, play a more important role in local virus amplification than larger species because they develop a higher, more persistent, viraemia.

EEE virus has been found in the northeastern and southeastern United States, primarily along coastal areas, and periodically in the upper Midwest, most recently in southwestern Michigan. Evidence of viral transmission in the bird-mosquito zoonotic cycle is usually detected in late spring and early summer to late fall (autumn) in recurrent foci of transmission.

As with most zoonotic infections, no apparent morbidity or mortality is observed in the natural hosts that become infected with EEE virus. Following the primary viral infection, an immunological response is detectable and persists for a protracted period. However, in some birds, including the Chukar (*Alectoris graeca*) (Moulthrop & Gordy 1960), House Sparrow (*Passer domesticus*) (Byrne et al. 1961), and Ring-necked Pheasant (*Phasianus colchicus*) (Sussman et al. 1958), that have been introduced into the USA, extensive mortality has been observed following an EEE viral infection. In this regard, the Whooping Crane deaths at PWRC in 1984 represent the first deaths associated with an EEE viral infection in an indigenous North American bird.

This unprecedented event has presented the US Fish and Wildlife Service, as part of its responsibilities for propagation and maintenance of the Whooping Crane, with an additional consideration that must be addressed in attempts to establish new populations. Successful establishment of new flocks would help to avert a single calamity that could further reduce Whooping Crane numbers (Kuyt 1976). However, if the reintroduction site proves to be an area with high EEE virus activity, Whooping Crane deaths could result. The three areas now under consideration were selected primarily because of habitat characteristics favourable to the Whooping Crane, without regard to EEE viral activity.

The first site is approximately 100km south of Orlando, Florida, in Osceola, Okeechobee, and Polk Counties. This area consists largely of agricultural fields. Although evidence of EEE virus transmission has been identified throughout much of Florida, the areas of greatest endemicity are north of the proposed site (Bigler et al. 1975; Bigler et al. 1976). The second site is a marshy area adjacent to the Okefenokee Swamp in Georgia. Both of these reintroductions are likely to result in nonmigratory flocks. Studies conducted in southeastern Georgia, just north of the swamp, have revealed a long history of EEE viral infections in horses (Chamberlain et al. 1969). The mosquito *Culiseta melanura* is abundant in this locality and has yielded large numbers of EEE virus isolates. The third proposed reintroduction site is the Seney National Wildlife Refuge in Michigan's Upper Peninsula. EEE viral transmission has not been reported from this site, but outbreaks of EEE have been reported in southwestern Michigan (Brown 1947; McLean et al. 1985). Birds reintroduced to this site would probably winter on the Texas Gulf Coast, where EEE contact is unlikely.

In general, the risk of acquiring an EEE viral infection in the proposed sites appears greatest in Georgia, less in Florida, and least likely in Michigan. Since EEE viral transmission is an annual occurrence in certain areas, it will be important to conduct a habitat analysis and survey for EEE virus and its vectors before selecting one or more of the proposed sites.

Techniques for monitoring potential EEE virus vectors are readily available. Mosquito surveys that yield the vector species previously mentioned would alert authorities to potential problems. Light traps, using dry ice as a carbon dioxide source, can effectively sample the mosquito fauna. Mosquitoes can be collected, identified, and assayed for EEE virus. Studies of the antibody prevalence to EEE virus in wild birds and/or sentinel birds in bird-baited traps would complement mosquito vector surveys. Simple, reliable, rapid diagnostic procedures are currently being developed to aid in these surveys (Scott & Olson 1986).

The results of vaccination suggest that this will afford protection to seronegative Whooping Cranes that are 'at risk' to a natural EEE viral infection. Unfortunately, routine administration of the inactivated EEE virus vaccine to wild Whooping Cranes is probably not practicable.

Because of the endangered status of the Whooping Crane, definitive laboratory experiments required to assess the efficacy of EEE virus vaccine have not been conducted. However, by monitoring antibody titres in vaccinated cranes in the spring and fall, it may be possible to detect an increase in antibody titres that would be expected following natural infection without clinical disease. Thus, a 'natural' challenge with EEE virus would provide a positive indication of the protective qualities of the vaccine.

In conclusion, the loss of seven captive Whooping Cranes to EEE virus in 1984 presented a previously unrecognized risk and obstacle to the species' recovery. Not only was there a setback in the captive breeding programme for the Whooping Crane, but, because of the susceptibility of the species to the EEE virus, establishment of additional crane populations may be more complicated than initially envisaged. However, with continued collaboration and support from concerned individuals and agencies, we are confident that the impact of EEE virus on Whooping Crane recovery can be overcome to the ultimate benefit of this endangered species.

ACKNOWLEDGEMENTS

We are grateful to Dr F. Joshua Dein, Patuxent Wildlife Research Center, U.S. Fish and Wildlife Service, Laurel, Maryland, for technical assistance throughout all phases of this study. Assistance from personnel at the following agencies is also gratefully acknowledged: National Wildlife Health Laboratory, U.S. Fish and Wildlife Service, Madison, Wisconsin, U.S. Army Medical Research Institute of Infectious Diseases, Ft. Detrick, Maryland; Maryland Department of Agriculture, Maryland; Department of the Army, U.S. Army Environmental Hygiene Agency, Ft. George G. Meade, Maryland; and, Department of Entomology, University of Maryland, College Park, Maryland.

REFERENCES

ALLEN, R. P. 1952. *The Whooping Crane*. Research Report 3. National Audubon Society, New York.
BIGLER, W. J., LASSING, E., BUFF, E., LEWIS, A. L. & HOFF, G. L. 1975. Arbovirus surveillance in Florida: wild vertebrate studies 1965–1974. *J. Wildl. Dis.* **11**: 348–56.
BIGLER, W. J., LASSING, E. B., BUFF, E. E., PRATHER, E. C., BECK, E. C. & HOFF, G. L. 1976. Endemic eastern equine encephalomyelitis in Florida: a twenty-year analysis, 1955–1974. *Am. J. Trop. Med. Hyg.* **25**: 884–90.
BROWN, G. C. 1947. Studies on equine encephalomyelitis in Michigan. *J. Infect. Dis.* **81**: 48–54.
BYRNE, R. J., HETRICK, F. M., SCANLON, J. E., HASTINGS, J. W. & LOCKE, L. N. 1961.

Observations on eastern equine encephalitis in Maryland in 1959. *J. Am. Vet. Med. Ass.* **139**: 661–4.

CARPENTER, J. W., DEIN, F. J. & CLARK, G. 1987. An outbreak of eastern equine encephalitis virus in captive whooping cranes. *Proceedings of the 1985 Crane Workshop, Grande Island, Nebraska.* Platte River Whooping Crane Habitat Maintenance Trust and U.S. Fish and Wildlife Service, Grande Island, Nebraska.

CHAMBERLAIN, R. W., SUDIA, W. D., COLEMAN, P. H., JOHNSTON, J. G. & WORK, T. H. 1969. Arbovirus isolations from mosquitoes collected in Waycross, Georgia, 1963, during an outbreak of equine encephalitis. *Am. J. Epidemiol.* **89**: 82–8.

CLARK, G. G., DEIN, F. J., CRABBS, C. L., CARPENTER, J. W. & WATTS, D. M. 1987. Antibody response of sandhill and whooping cranes to an eastern equine encephalitis (EEE) virus vaccine. *J. Wildlife Dis.* **23**: 539–44.

DEIN, F. J., CARPENTER, J. W., CLARK, G. G., MONTALI, R. J., CRABBS, C. L., TSAI, T. F. & DOCHERTY, D. E. 1986. Mortality of captive whooping cranes caused by eastern equine encephalitis virus. *J. Am. Vet. Med. Ass.* **189**: 1006–10.

ERICKSON, R. C. 1968. A federal research program for endangered wildlife. *Trans. N. Amer. Wildl. Conf.* **33**: 418–33.

ERICKSON, R. C. & DERRICKSON, S. R. 1981. The whooping crane. *In:* Lewis, J. C. & Masatomi, H. (eds). *Crane Research Around the World.* Proc. Internat. Crane Symp. Sapporo, Japan, in 1980, and papers from World Working Group on Cranes, ICBP.

KISSLING, R. E., CHAMBERLAIN, R. W., SIKES, R. K. & EDISON, M. E. 1954. Studies on the North American encephalitides. III. Eastern equine encephalitis in wild birds. *Am. J. Hyg.* **60**: 251–65.

KUYT, E. 1976. Whooping cranes: the long road back. *Natur. Can.* **5**: 2–9.

MCLEAN, R. M., FRIER, G., PARHAM, G. L., FRANCY, D. B., MONATH, T. P., CAMPOS, E. G., THERRIEN, A., KERSCHNER, J. & CALISHER, C. H. 1985. Investigations of the vertebrate hosts of eastern equine encephalitis during an epizootic in Michigan, 1980. *Am. J. Trop. Med. Hyg.* **34**: 1190–1202.

MOULTHROP, I. M. & GORDY, B. A. 1960. Eastern viral encephalomyelitis in chukar (*Alectoris graeca*). *Avian Dis.* **4**: 380–3.

SCOTT, T. W. & OLSON, J. G. 1986. Detection of eastern equine encephalomyelitis viral antigen in avian blood by enzyme immunoassay: a laboratory study. *Am. J. Trop. Med. Hyg.* **35**: 611–18.

STAMM, D. D. 1963. Susceptibility of bird populations to eastern, western, and St. Louis encephalitis viruses. *Proc. Intl. Ornithol. Congr.* **13**: 591–603.

SUSSMAN, O., COHEN, D., GERENDE, J. E. & KISSLING, R. E. 1958. Equine encephalitis vaccine studies in pheasants under epizootic and preepizootic conditions. *Ann. N.Y. Acad. Sci.* **70**: 328–41.

U.S. FISH AND WILDLIFE SERVICE. 1986. *Whooping Crane Recovery Plan.* U.S. Fish and Wildlife Service, Albuquerque, New Mexico.

WILLIAMS, J. E., WATTS, D. M., YOUNG, O. P. & REED, T. J. 1972. Transmission of eastern (EEE) and western (WEE) encephalitis to bobwhite sentinels in relation to density of *Culiseta melanura* mosquitoes. *Mosq. News* **32**: 188–92.

THE ROLE OF BIRDS IN THE LONG-DISTANCE DISPERSAL OF DISEASE

W. R. P. BOURNE

Department of Zoology, Aberdeen University, Tillydrone Avenue, Aberdeen AB9 2TN, Scotland

ABSTRACT

Birds can play an important role in the dissemination of organisms of various kinds. Pathogens can be transported mechanically, or the bird may be a biological vector. An historic incident which has escaped documentation hitherto is reported. A strain of influenza appeared in a flock of chickens kept next to a seabird colony in Scotland at a time of active bird migration. The virus isolated was subsequently found to share an antigen with another strain of influenza which shortly afterwards caused mortality among Common Terns (*Sterna hirundo*) in their winter quarters in South Africa. There is a need for a more concerted and multidisciplinary approach to the study of such incidents, and for the application of research to the management and protection of threatened species.

DEDICATION

This contribution is dedicated to the memory of Dr Harry Hoogstraal (1917–1986), a tireless investigator and helpful colleague who made a vast contribution to a major branch of the subject, the relation between birds, ticks, and disease, during 37 years of service with the Department of Medical Zoology of United States Naval Medical Research Unit No. 3, in Cairo, Egypt. Although it was hoped that he might help provide a larger contribution, he died earlier in the year in which this paper was prepared. His work lives on at a new Center for Tick Research, named after him, at the United States National Museum. The Center contains the largest collection and library in the world devoted to the subject.

INTRODUCTION

Birds are susceptible to infectious and parasitic diseases similar to those affecting other animals, and are chiefly notable from this point of view because their mobility confers upon them an unusually important role in the long-distance dispersal of many organisms. It must be borne in mind that every autumn over five thousand million birds migrate from the Western and Central Palearctic to their wintering areas in Africa. This is a vast subject involving tens of thousands of references, a small selection of which are listed at the end of this paper.

The success of living organisms is limited by their ability to colonize new habitats and to survive the natural hazards, or in the case of other organisms defences, that they encounter there. Birds provide a promising field for such parasitism because they are numerous and widespread, with vulnerable plumage and nest-sites, and are often sociable, mobile, and liable to prey upon each other in ways that assist the dispersal of accompanying organisms. Although important where they occur, such opportunities for dispersal may not, however, arise very often, so that bird parasites must also develop an unusual capacity for direct dispersal, extreme powers of endurance, or the ability to make use of alternative hosts, which the birds either eat, (e.g. the worms infesting aquatic animals) or which feed upon the birds (e.g. various blood-sucking arthropods). Certain more complex forms may move about themselves at some stage in their life-cycle, and also make use of a succession of hosts, some of which may also be themselves parasites.

This obscure subject, which is difficult to study and presents little attraction for the casual observer, is of importance both as a major factor limiting bird numbers, which may become particularly serious when the birds are already under stress for other reasons (Cooper, this volume; Thomson 1961; Herman 1969) and because it may affect human health and husbandry (Keymer 1974; Bourne 1975), and therefore public attitudes to birds. Thus, for example, while birds are often accused of transmitting foot-and-mouth disease, it appears to be spread much more often over short distances by the wind (Murton 1964; Donaldson 1983) and over longer ones in meat products, so that the authorities should not be allowed to blame birds without stronger evidence than they can usually supply for outbreaks of this disease.

Similarly, although all the birds in the neighbourhood were slaughtered along with other more likely vectors after one outbreak of rabies in Britain, there is much less public awareness of the more serious risk of the transport of avian disease by cagebirds (Ashton 1984; Keymer 1974; Laird & Hoogstraal 1975; Alexander *et al.* 1977), which provides one of the strongest arguments against this trade. Pathogenic organisms can also be carried from one country to another by birds that are being transported to or from captive breeding programmes: these may either be threatened species themselves or foster birds (Cooper, this volume).

Birds may transport micro-organisms in a variety of ways, and this subject is discussed in detail elsewhere (Reece, this volume). In this paper an example is used to illustrate the problems that may occur: the instance in question occurred thirty years ago but has not previously been properly documented. I am indebted to Dr H. G. Pereira at the National Institute for Medical Research, Mill Hill, London, and Professor G. M. Dunnet of Aberdeen University, for details.

BACKGROUND

'Fowl pest' is a descriptive term applied in Britain to a syndrome, often causing high mortality, which is now known to be caused by two distinct myxoviruses carried by wild birds (Bourne 1971). In wild birds they vary greatly in virulence (McFerran *et al.* 1968), though captive stocks kept under unnatural conditions appear to be more susceptible. Classical 'fowl plague', which was first recorded in Italy in 1878, and is now known to be caused by various strains of Influenza

A also circulating in mammals, including man and his domestic animals (Kaplan & Beveridge 1972), was until recently seldom detected in birds. This is possibly because it spreads mainly by direct contact when the birds huddle together in roosts, or when waterbirds dabble in each others' faeces, and often fails to kill wild birds. In contrast an allied disease, first distinguished in Newcastle-upon-Tyne in 1926, and therefore named after that town, which apparently causes its most marked effects in birds, may also be spread by the wind (Smith 1964), resulting in endless problems for the poultry industry (Allan 1971), although it should be noted that it can also cause a mild lacrimal infection in humans and is therefore classified as a zoonosis (Anon 1984).

The outbreak of avian influenza with which the author had a marginal connection, and which has not been properly documented, occurred in an area of mixed farming near the northeast coast of Scotland in 1959. Becker (1966) has postulated that the disease may first have caused the deaths of numbers of Fulmars (*Fulmarus glacialis*) and Kittiwakes (*Rissa tridactyla*) washed ashore by the prevailing west winds on the far side of the North Sea during the summer (Joensen 1959). In the course of observations with radar in the vicinity of the vast seabird breeding colonies frequented by these species north of Aberdeen during the following autumn, an unusually prolonged spell of east winds in October transported exceptional numbers of all sorts of disorientated and drifted continental landbird migrants, especially thrushes, west across the North Sea, so that thousands of exhausted birds remained feeding around the farms near the shore for weeks (Bourne 1963). Many of these birds, any of which might have been infected, are likely to have been consumed by the innumerable local Herring Gulls (*Larus argentatus*) and infected them, but the latter tend to be resistant to viruses (McFerran et al. 1968) and appeared to remain healthy.

The Herring Gulls, which attract attention because they steal food put out for stock, were noticed to frequent a farm about five kilometres inland from the coast throughout the summer, and it was doubtless also visited by the transient continental landbird migrants which tend to attract less attention in October. At the beginning of November, 250 one- and two-year-old domestic fowl and 14 ducks kept on free range were brought into a deep litter house for the winter. After about a fortnight the fowl began to die, and approximately one hundred were lost over the next six weeks, after which the losses ceased. During the early stages of the outbreak the birds were in good condition and laying, and died suddenly, or were found dead, often in the nestboxes, without having shown any signs of illness. Later cases became dull and listless, with pale combs which had cyanosed tips, and almost all showed marked oedema of the face, wattles and submandibular space. They took 12–36 hours to die, with the deaths evenly divided between the two age-groups. There appeared to be no difference between breeds (strains) of bird.

The outbreak was reported to the Ministry of Agriculture, Fisheries and Food Veterinary Laboratory at Lasswade, Scotland, where it was investigated by Dr J. E. Wilson. The bodies showed the classical lesions of fowl plague, and a distinct strain of Influenza A was isolated, which proved lethal for poultry although it had little effect on wild birds, including Herring Gulls. Two other groups of fowl kept in adjacent deep litter houses remained healthy, and no other abnormal bird mortality was noticed in the area, which the author was surveying daily at the time in ignorance of the outbreak. Subsequently the surviving poultry were also investigated, but none still carried the virus, named 'Influenza A/Chicken/Scotland/59', although about half the affected group had haemagglutination (HI) inhibition antibodies. It was never detected in birds from two adjacent litter houses or elsewhere in Scotland.

A similar incident involving a more virulent strain of influenza with the same haemagglutinin as the classical Dutch fowl plague of the 1920s, which resulted in the slaughter of 29,000 turkeys on a farm five kilometres inland from further large colonies of other seabirds off the north coast of Norfolk in southeast Britain in May 1963, led to the suggestion that this disease might be spread by wild birds on an intercontinental scale (Wells 1963). This hypothesis was supported by the discovery that a massive mortality of wintering European Common Terns (*Sterna hirundo*) around the coast of South Africa in April 1961 (Rowan 1962) was due to a strain of influenza with the same neuraminidase found in Scotland, duly named 'Influenza A/Tern/South Africa/1961' (Becker 1966). Although it is known from ringing/banding recoveries that the terns that breed within 16 kilometres of both outbreaks in Britain winter further north, and that the birds that were affected in the winter around South Africa breed around the Baltic, both populations, and indeed many other closely related terns which range from Arctic Canada and Siberia to the Antarctic, must mingle at roosts while on migration around the coast of West Africa.

DISCUSSION

While the evidence for involvement of wild birds in these outbreaks of disease in domestic fowl and turkeys must remain circumstantial, it appears probable that they were the source of the infection.

It is now recognized that many different strains of influenza A, characterized by the possession of variations of two distinct antigens, occur at intervals in many countries in wild populations of waterbirds, and also in seals, whales, and in at least one case Starlings (*Sturnus vulgaris*) (WHO 1981). Although their relationship to similar strains which periodically infect humans and domestic animals requires confirmation, it appears that each strain may circulate rapidly through the population of one or more species of animal in an area until a high proportion of the individuals develop an immunity to that particular strain, at which point it is replaced by another strain to which they have not yet developed an immunity. The original strain then moves on to another host or area for a period of years until the proportion of vulnerable individuals in the first host population starts to rise again.

It seems possible that for much of the time, birds are only involved in this process when they become infected with strains of influenza occurring in other animals. Formerly, birds were probably the main vehicle for dispersal of viruses over long distances until jet aircraft, which travel faster than birds and by varied routes, may have become more important. At the same time, changes in land-use—for example, the construction of man-made lakes or the planting of forests—may permit some pathogens to establish themselves or to spread (Pavlovsky 1966; Keast 1977). Incidents of the kind described are of interest because they provide a rare insight into complex biological processes which are sometimes of considerable epidemiological or economic importance, but which escape notice because of the highly specialized nature of the techniques, and scarcity of the resources, required to study them. This is a comparatively simple situation, involving the development of a parasitic micro-organism that has become sufficiently infectious to be spread easily between a variety of animals via the air and direct contact, and then has a sufficiently serious impact on the host to elicit the rapid development of immunity if it survives, countered by the development of variation in the parasite which enables it to evade the immune response. Thus, different strains of virus are able to circulate continually among different animal populations, some of which periodically prove lethal for some hosts, as with the strain of influenza found in domestic pigs which is believed to have caused more deaths among mankind in 1918 than the preceding World War.

The catalogue of organisms that may be spread by birds and can sometimes infect humans, livestock and crops is vast (Herman 1955). In recent years the role of migrating ducks in disseminating duck virus enteritis ('duck plague'), paramyxo- and other viruses has become increasingly recognized (Brand & Docherty 1984; Gough et al. 1987; Nerome et al. 1988), as has the probable part played by feral and other free-living pigeons in the maintenance and spread of avian paramyxovirus (Lister et al. 1986). Micro-organisms may present a threat to humans as well as to birds—for instance, *Chlamydia psittaci*, the cause of ornithosis or psittacosis (Keymer 1974; Wobeser & Brand 1982); bacteria of the genus *Salmonella*, often implicated in food-poisoning (Bourne 1977; Williams 1984); and the fungus *Histoplasma capsulatum*, responsible for histoplasmosis (Jackson 1973; Southern 1986; Tiffany et al. 1955; Warner & French 1970). Birds may also spread algae (Schlichting 1960), flowering plants (McAtee 1947), and many metazoan animals including leeches, helminths and arthropods. The organism concerned may remain entirely passive, so that its presence has comparatively little effect on the bird, as in the case of seeds or pathogens which are carried mechanically (for example, on the feet); in other cases it may become highly invasive and need to be able to move on in the event of the death of, or development of resistance by, its host.

One relatively simple method of dispersal of pathogens occurs when the organism makes use of biting insects (especially Diptera) which are often associated with birds. Many protozoa are spread in this way (Peirce, this volume). However, this has the disadvantage that the insect vectors seldom live long or travel far, so that the method only provides a temporary expedient in areas where hosts are numerous. In other cases, such as that of the arboviruses where hosts are scarce or local and it may be necessary to wait a long time (sometimes at least a season) to find one, insects prove less satisfactory vectors. In such instances arachnids such as ticks or mites, which wait long periods for hosts to come to them (but also hitch an occasional intercontinental lift themselves—Hoogstraal et al. 1961) may prove more satisfactory. The infection that is transmitted may or may not cause clinical disease in the host in addition to the direct effect of the ticks themselves (Duffy & Duffy 1986; Schilling et al. 1981; Hoogstraal et al. 1970–82). Thus, for example, one bite by an immature arbovirus-carrying tick *Ornithodoros meusebecki* on Zirqa Island in the lower Persian (Arabian) Gulf in December 1972 led to immediate swelling and a persistent nodule at the site of the bite, and was followed within hours by a period of fever and delirium lasting some two days (John Stewart-Smith, pers. comm.). Nearly every recorded encounter with this tick has been followed by the development of sores at the site of the bite (Hoogstraal & Gallagher 1982), and there is always a risk of potentially fatal encephalitis, one reason for discouraging unnecessary disturbance to colonies of colonial birds.

Perhaps the most spectacular technique utilized by pathogenic micro-organisms is that illustrated by *Clostridium botulinum*. This bacterium multiplies anaerobically in decaying matter, where it secretes one of the most toxic poisons known. It kills more potential food and is then passed on to further victims in the resulting maggots, until the supply fails, when the organism forms spores which can remain dormant for long periods or be carried on the feet of surviving prey to infect new habitats (Smith 1976; Lloyd *et al.* 1976; Wobeser 1981). Many other organisms can also be transported on the integument (feet, feathers, skin) of birds: examples include bacteria of the species *Staphylococcus aureus, Escherichia coli* and *Clostridium tetani*, resistant forms of certain parasites (helminth ova and coccidial oocysts) and certain viruses e.g. avian pox. Potential pathogens can also be carried mechanically in the alimentary tract, but the gut transit time of birds tends to be short (Cooper 1987), so the chances of long-distance dispersal by this means are slight.

Perhaps the most effective way of spreading a pathogen on a large scale is for the hosts (birds) to become infected with the organism and thus maintain its viability. This appears to be the case with some of the viruses, as the examples related earlier show, and the results can be spectacular. As other chapters in this book emphasize, it is important that every opportunity is taken to examine and take samples from wild birds that are found dead or dying or even appear healthy but may be harbouring micro-organisms. The screening of birds on migration—for example, when they are being ringed/banded—can provide particularly valuable information (Cooper 1989). It is particularly important to keep watch for sick birds that drop out of migrations or appear in consignments of cage birds, and for infection spreading into any bird populations that come into contact with them, as in the cases discussed initially.

There can be no doubt that the role of wild birds in the dissemination of disease needs more careful study. The literature on the subject tends to be scattered, and people from different disciplines are often involved. A concerted approach, involving ornithologists, wildlife biologists, veterinarians, physicians and public health officials, could help to elucidate some of the problems. At the same time, the actual and potential impact of infectious and parasitic disease on threatened bird populations, both in the wild and in captivity, could be assessed.

REFERENCES

ALEXANDER, D. J., ALLAN, W. H. & SILLARS, T. 1977. Isolation of myxoviruses from dead birds arriving at Heathrow Airport, London. *J. Hyg. Camb.* **79**: 243–7.

ALLAN, W. H. 1971. The problem of Newcastle Disease. *Nature* **234**: 129–31.

ANON, 1984. Newcastle Disease. U.S. Department of Agriculture. *Program Aid No. 1092.* U.S. Government Printing Office.

ASHTON, W. L. G. 1984. The risks and problems connected with the import and export of captive birds. *Br. Vet. J.* **140**: 317–27.

BECKER, W. B. 1966. The isolation and classification of Tern virus: Influenza Virus A/Tern/South Africa/1961. *J. Hyg. Camb.* **64**: 309–20.

BOURNE, W. R. P. 1963. *Bird Migration in Scotland studied by Radar.* Manuscript deposited with the Edward Grey Institute, Oxford, Aberdeen University Library, British Trust for Ornithology and Scottish Ornithologists' Club.

BOURNE, W. R. P. 1971. Influenza virus reappears. *BTO News* **44**: 4.

BOURNE, W. R. P. 1975. Birds and hazards to health. *Practitioner* **215**: 165–71.

BOURNE, W. R. P. 1977. Seabirds and *Salmonella. Mar. Pollut. Bull.* **8**: 194–5.

BRAND, C. J. & DOCHERTY, D. E. 1984. A survey of North American migratory waterfowl for duck plague (duck virus enteritis) virus. *J. Wildl. Dis.* **20**: 261–6.

COOPER, J. E. 1987. Introduction to birds. *In:* Poole, T. B. (ed.). *The UFAW Handbook on the Care and Management of Laboratory Animals.* Longman, Essex.

COOPER, J. E. 1989. The importance of health monitoring of migrating raptors. *Proceedings of the III World Conference on Birds of Prey.* March 1987, Israel.

DONALDSON, A. I. 1983. Quantitative data on airborne foot-and-mouth disease virus: its production, carriage and deposition. *In:* Brooksby, J. B. The Aerial Transmission of Disease. *Trans. R. Soc. Lond.* **B 302**: 529–34.

DUFFY, D. C. & DUFFY M. J. C. D. 1986. Tick parasitism at nesting colonies of blue-footed boobies in Peru and Galapagos. *Condor* **88**: 242–4.

GOUGH, R. E., BORLAND, E. O., KEYMER, I. F. & STUART, J. C. 1987. An outbreak of duck virus enteritis in commercial ducks and geese in East Anglia. *Vet. Rec.* **121**: 85.

HERMAN, C. M. 1955. Diseases of birds. *Recent Studies in Avian Biology*, 450–67. University of Illinois Press, Urbana.

HERMAN, C. M. 1969. The impact of disease on wildlife populations. *Bioscience* **19**: 321–5, 330.

HOOGSTRAAL, H., GALIN, A. L. & DJIGOUNIAN, A. 1970–82. *Bibliography of Ticks and Tick-born Diseases from Homer (about 800BC) to 31 December 1981*. 7 vols. United States Medical Research Unit No. 3 Special Publications, Cairo, Egypt.

HOOGSTRAAL, H. & GALLAGHER, M. D. 1982. Blisters, pruritus and fever after bites by the Arabian tick *Ornithodoros (Alectorobius) muesebecki. Lancet* **2**: 288–9.

HOOGSTRAAL, H., KAISER, M. N. & TRAYLOR, M. A. 1961. Ticks (Ixodidae) on birds migrating from Africa to Europe and Asia. *Bull. Wld. Hlth. Org.* **24**: 197–212.

JACKSON, J. A. 1973. Histoplasmosis—an occupational hazard for bird-banders? *IBBA News* **45**: 52–7.

JOENSEN, A. H. 1959. Disaster among fulmars (*Fulmarus glacialis*) and kittiwakes (*Rissa tridactyla*) in Danish waters in 1959. *Dansk Orn. Foren. Tidsskr.* **55**: 212–18.

KAPLAN, M. & BEVERIDGE, W. I. B. (eds). 1972. Influenza in animals. *Bull. Wld. Hlth. Org.* **47**: 439–42.

KEAST, D. 1977. Avian parasites and infectious disease. *Emu* **77**: 188–92.

KEYMER, I. F. 1974. Ornithosis in free-living and captive birds. *Proc. Roy. Soc. Med.* **67**: 733–5.

LAIRD, M. & HOOGSTRAAL, H. 1975. Disease hazards associated with bird importations. *Environ. Conserv.* **2**: 119–20.

LISTER, S. A., ALEXANDER, D. J. & HOGG, R. A. 1986. Evidence for the presence of avian paramyxovirus type I in feral pigeons in England and Wales. *Vet. Rec.* **118**: 476–9.

LLOYD, C. S., THOMAS, G. J., MACDONALD, J. W., BORLAND, E. D., STANLEY, K. D. & SMART, J. L. 1976. Wild bird mortality caused by botulism in Britain in 1975. *Biol. Conserv.* **10**: 119–29.

MCATEE, W. L. 1947. Distribution of seeds by birds. *Amer. Midl. Natur.* **38**: 214–23.

MCFERRAN, J. B., GORDON, W. A. M. & FINLAY, J. T. T. 1968. An outbreak of subclinical Newcastle Disease in Northern Ireland. *Vet. Rec.* **82**: 589–92.

MURTON, R. K. 1964. Do birds transmit foot and mouth disease? *Ibis* **106**: 289–98.

NEROME, K., ISHIDA, M. MATSUMATO, M. & ABE, K. 1988. Paramyxovirus isolated from migrating ducks. *In:* Darai, G. (ed.). *Virus Disease in Laboratory and Captive Animals*. Martinus Nijhoff, Boston.

PAVLOVSKY, E. N. 1966. *Natural Nidality of Transmissible Diseases*, English translation. University of Illinois Press, Urbana and London.

ROWAN, M. K. 1962. Mass mortality among European Common Terns in South Africa in April–May 1961. *Brit. Birds* **55**: 103–14.

SCHILLING, F., BÖTTCHER, M. & WALTER, G. 1981. Probleme des Zeckenbefalls bei Nestlingen des Wanderfalken (*Falco peregrinus*). *J. Orn.* **122**: 359–67.

SCHLICHTING, H. E. 1960. The role of waterfowl in the dispersal of algae. *Trans. Amer. Microsc. Soc.* **79**: 160–66.

SMITH, C. V. 1964. Some evidence for the wind-borne spread of fowl pest. *Met. Mag.* **93**: 257–63.

SMITH, G. R. 1976. Botulism in waterfowl. *Wildfowl* **27**: 129–38.

SOUTHERN, W. E. 1986. Commentary: Histoplasmosis associated with a gull colony: health and precautions. *Colon. Waterbirds* **9**: 121–3.

THOMSON, H. V. 1961. Ecology of diseases in wild mammals and birds. *Vet. Rec.* **73**: 1334–7.

TIFFANY, L. H., GILMAN, J. C. & MURPHY, D. F. 1955. Fungi from birds associated with wilted oaks in Iowa. *Iowa State Coll. J. Sci.* **29**: 659–706.
WARNER, G.M. & FRENCH, D. W. 1970. Dissemination of fungi by migrating birds: survival and recovery of fungi from birds. *Can. J. Bot.* **48**: 907–10.
WELLS, R. J. H. 1963. An outbreak of fowl plague in turkeys. *Vet. Rec.* **75**: 783–6.
WHO 1981. The ecology of influenza viruses: a WHO Memorandum. *Bull. Wld Hlth Org.* **59**: 869–73.
WILLIAMS, J. E. 1984. Paratyphoid infections. *In:* Hofstad, M. S., Barnes, H. J., Calnek, B. W., Reid, W. M. & Yoder, H. W. (eds). *Diseases of Poultry* 8th edition. Iowa State University Press, Ames.
WOBESER, G. A. 1981. *Diseases of Wild Waterfowl.* Plenum Press, New York.
WOBESER, G. & BRAND, C. J. 1982. Chlamydiosis in two biologists investigating disease occurrences in wild waterfowl. *Wildl. Soc. Bull.* **10**: 170–2.

FURTHER READING

ALEXANDER, D. J. & GOUGH, R. E. 1986. Isolations of avian influenza virus from birds in Great Britain. *Vet. Rec.* **118**: 537–8.
ALEXANDER, D. J., MACKENZIE, J. S. & RUSSELL, P. H. 1986. Two types of Newcastle disease viruses isolated from feral birds in Western Australia detected by monoclonal antibodies. *Aust. Vet. J.* **63**: 365–7.
ANON 1984. *Avian Influenza. A Threat to U.S. Poultry. Program Aid no. 1353.* U.S. Government Printing Office.
FRIEND, M. J. 1987. (ed.). *Field Guide to Wildlife Diseases. Volume 1.* General Field Procedures and Diseases of Migrating Birds. U.S. Department of the Interior. Fish and Wildlife Service, Washington D.C.
HALVORSON, D. A., KELLEHERC, J. & SENNE, D. A. 1985. Epizootiology of avian influenza: effect of season on incidence in sentinel ducks and domestic turkeys in Minnesota. *Appl. Environ. Microb.* **49**: 914–19.
LIPKIND, M., RIVETZ, B. & SHIHMANTER, E. 1987. The first isolation of Newcastle disease virus (NDV) from free-flying birds in Israel: comparative studies on NDV strain isolated from migrating starlings (*Sturnus vulgaris*) wintering in Israel. *Comp. Immunol. Microbiol. Infect. Dis.* **10**: 65–70.
ROBERTSON, D. G. 1981. The disease threat to Australia from migrating birds. *In:* Fowler, M. E. (ed.). *Wildlife Diseases of the Pacific Basin and other Countries.* Wildlife Disease Association.

MONITORING PARASITES IN WILD AND CAPTIVE GREEN PEAFOWL IN THAILAND

N. Hillgarth[1], C. C. Norton[2], M. A. Peirce[3] & B. Stewart Cox[4]

1 Department of Zoology, Oxford University, South Parks Road, Oxford OX1 3PS, England.
2 Ministry of Agriculture, Fisheries and Food, Central Veterinary Laboratory, New Haw, Weybridge, Surrey KT15 3NB, England.
3 16 Westmorland Close, Woosehill, Wokingham, Berkshire RG11 9AZ, England.
4 c/o D3 Praphai House, Soi Pattana Sin, Nang Linchee Road, Bangkok 10120, Thailand.

ABSTRACT

Faecal samples were collected from wild (free-living) Green Peafowl (*Pavo muticus*) in Huai Kha Kheng Wildfowl Sanctuary in Thailand and examined for parasites. Faeces and blood smears were also collected from captive peafowl. The wild peafowl showed low levels of four types of coccidial oocysts and a few helminth ova. Blood smears from one wild bird contained a haemoproteid parasite. The captive birds showed even lower parasite levels. The implications for captive breeding and release programmes are discussed.

INTRODUCTION

The Blue Peafowl (*Pavo cristatus*) from the Indian sub-continent must be one of the most familiar birds in the world. Today there are a great number of these birds in parks and zoos, and feral populations have been established in areas as diverse as South America, Australia and Europe.

The Green Peafowl (*Pavo muticus*), however, though much admired in its native Asia, has always been less well known elsewhere. The Green Peafowl has an upright, pointed crest, and a longer neck and legs than the Blue. The overall plumage is similar except that the feathers have a broad metallic border, giving the bird a very bright appearance. A striking difference between the two species is that the Green female has a bright plumage similar to that of the full adult male, but without the long train.

The Green Peafowl is now an endangered species. Once it was found throughout Southeast Asia, southern China and Indonesia. During the past twenty years its range has been drastically reduced and it is now thought to occur only in parts of western Burma, central Thailand, southern China on the Vietnamese border, Kampuchea (Cambodia) and Java. The populations in each known area are very small, and it is estimated that there are only between 1000 and 2000 birds left in the wild. There are also about 500 birds in captivity, many of which are in Thailand (Hillgarth & Stewart Cox 1986).

The Oxford Green Peafowl Project in Thailand was established in co-operation with the Thai Forestry Department and supported by many organisations in Britain and Thailand. Its aims are to study the Green Peafowl's biology in an effort to understand the reasons for the species' dramatic decline, and to provide a foundation for future management. One of the aims of the study was to determine the presence and possible significance of parasitic infection, and to establish if there was any potential threat to free-living birds should infected captive peafowl be released back into the wild. In addition, other (pheasant) species were sampled.

MATERIALS AND METHODS

A preliminary investigation was carried out from January to March 1986 in the Huai Kha Kheng Wildlife Sanctuary, 200km north of Bangkok, in an area of bamboo and mixed deciduous forest bisected by a river of the same name. This is the last stronghold of Green Peafowl in Thailand. There are no more than 200 peafowl in the area, living in proximity to the river and its tributaries.

In addition, two government pheasant captive breeding centres and three private collections were visited. Fresh faecal samples were collected from 38 peafowl and 17 pheasants and preserved in two percent potassium dichromate. These were examined for coccidial oocysts and helminth eggs by standard methods, including flotation methods using a McMasters' slide, and oocysts that sporulated were measured and described (MAFF 1977). Blood smears were prepared according to the method of Peirce & Prince (1980). Ectoparasites were collected and preserved in 70 percent alcohol.

RESULTS

Wild (free-living) Green Peafowl

The study area included ten kilometres of river and an estimated 25 peafowl. They display and feed on the sandbanks of the river, and their faeces are easy to collect because they are large and round and unlike those of any other animals in the area. Fourteen fresh samples were collected, eight of which were from individual adult birds observed defaecating and six from separate areas which were probably from different birds.

Coccidia and helminth ova recovered from these samples are recorded in *Table 1*. Half the dichromate-preserved samples contained sufficient material to count the coccidial oocysts; the remainder were examined by a salt-flotation concentration technique. The numbers of oocysts per gramme of faeces were relatively low and two samples were negative.

Four types of oocysts were seen (*Table 1*). Type A were subspherical and measured 15.1–17.7μm × 13.9–14.5μm; mean 16.7 × 14.3μm. A polar granule was present. The ellipsoidal sporocysts possessed two large sporozoite globules. Type B were ellipsoidal with a colourless oocyst wall and an indistinct micropyle. They measured 22.1–23.3μm × 16.5–19.6μm; mean 22.9 × 18.7μm. A single polar granule was present. Sporocysts were asymmetrical with one straight side, and measured 12.8 × 6.5μm. Type C oocysts were dark yellow in colour, ovoid

Table 1: Coccidia and helminths in faeces from wild Green Peafowl in Huai Kha Kheng Wildlife Sanctuary, Thailand.

Bird No.	Known bird	Oocysts Per g	A	B	C	D	Helminth ova
1	Yes	2200	55	45	—	—	—
2	Yes	3600	46	—	54	—	—
3	Yes	3400	—	35	65	—	—
4	Yes	800	—	—	100	—	—
5	Yes	7400	19	61	20	—	Very few
6	Yes	1300	14	64	22	—	Very few
7	Yes	4800	16	84	—	—	—
8	Yes	Numerous	17	74	—	9	—
9	No	Very few	44	16	40	—	—
10	No	Few	—	41	59	—	—
11	No	Few	17	58	25	—	Very few
12	No	0	—	—	—	—	—
13	No	Few	42	27	31	—	—
14	No	0	—	—	—	—	—

in shape, and measured 26.5–27.1µm × 19.0µm; mean 26.8 × 19.0µm. One or two polar granules were present and the sporocysts were asymmetrical with one straight side. Type D oocysts occurred in a single bird and did not sporulate, but were distinguished from the others by their elongate ovoid shape.

Small numbers of helminth ova, too few for a count, occurred in three birds only (*Table 1*). These were not identified but appeared to be of the trichostrongyle-type in birds 5, 6 and 11, plus heterakid-type ova in birds 6 and 11. Blood smears obtained from a single wild Green Peafowl showed a haemoproteid red cell parasite, probably *Haemoproteus rileyi*. This bird had many ticks on the head and neck: the specimens are awaiting identification.

Captive peafowl and pheasants

Faecal samples from thirteen captive Green Peafowl at the Chonburi and Chantaburi pheasant breeding centres were negative for coccidia. Two samples contained a few ova of a *Capillaria* species. There was no history of treatment of these birds.

Of 11 samples from captive Green Peafowl held in three private collections, three were negative, seven contained a few oocysts of Types A, B and C, whilst a single juvenile bird showed numerous oocysts of Type A. No helminth ova were seen in these samples. A sample from a single Blue Peafowl contained a few degenerate oocysts which resembled Types A, B and C from the Green Peafowl.

Faecal samples from 17 individual birds of five different pheasant species were collected from the breeding centre at Chantaburi. Twelve of these were negative, but those from a Crested Fireback (*Lophura ignita*) and a Siamese Fireback (*Lophura diardi*) contained a few ovoid oocysts. A second Siamese Fireback sample contained a few broadly ellipsoidal oocysts with a light brown, punctate wall. An Argus Pheasant (*Argusianus argus*) had a few small subspherical oocysts.

Blood smears were obtained from nine captive Green Peafowl, one Blue Peafowl, one Jungle Fowl (*Gallus* sp.) and one Lady Amherst Pheasant (*Chrysolophus amherstiae*). A Rickettsia-like organism was found in four Green Peafowl and the single Blue Peafowl. One Green Peafowl had a chronic infection with a *Plasmodium* species, but the absence of mature gametocytes or schizonts made a definitive identification impossible. A low parasitaemia with a leucocytozoon, probably *Leucocytozoon caulleryi*, was present in the Jungle Fowl.

DISCUSSION

Wild (free-living) Green Peafowl at Huai Kha Kheng showed a low level of parasitic infection. The number of coccidial oocysts per gramme of faeces was consistent with the level of infection seen in adult wild birds of other gallinaceous species (Bejsovec 1972).

The material provided insufficient data for a specific identification of the various oocyst types. No coccidia have been described previously from the Green Peafowl. Those described from the Blue Peafowl in India (Pellérdy 1974) may or may not be shared between the two hosts. The oocysts designated Type A resembled those of *Eimeria pavonis* Mandal, 1960, but possessed no oocyst residuum. The asymmetrical sporocysts observed in Types B and C do not correspond to any of the coccidia from the Blue Peafowl, and it seems likely that these are hitherto undescribed species.

Eimeria mayurai (Bhatia & Pande 1966) and *Isospora mayurai* (Patnaik 1966) are pathogenic in the Blue Peafowl. The pathogenicity of coccidia in the Green Peafowl is not known and could best be established by examination of juveniles in the wild and by experimental infection of captive birds.

Assessing the impact of coccidial infection on wild populations is difficult. It is generally assumed that coccidiosis occurs less frequently in the wild than in captivity where birds are often raised in more crowded conditions. In Czechoslovakia, Bejsovec (1972, 1977a) assessed the effect of coccidia on wild gamebird populations by carrying out extensive faecal examinations. He concluded that coccidial infection was not responsible for the long-term fluctuation in pheasant and partridge populations which accompanied the changes in landscape following the introduction of large-scale farming. Coccidia persisted in relict populations of Capercaillie (*Tetrao urogallus*) and Black Grouse (*Lyrurus tetrix*) in Czechoslovakia (Bejsovec 1977b, 1979). The concentration of birds for mating and subsequent chick rearing, and the extent of infection recorded at this time, suggested that coccidia might cause a further decline in the population of these birds. In all these studies, the relation between the oocysts recorded in the faeces and actual disease in the host is not clear. In pheasants, however, coccidiosis was found in 82 percent of the dead chicks examined (Bejsovec 1978).

The potential danger of coccidiosis in captive breeding for subsequent release into the wild is exemplified by the reports of disseminated visceral coccidiosis in the Sandhill Crane (*Grus canadensis*), used to hatch the chicks of the endangered Whooping Crane (*Grus americana*) (Carpenter et al. 1980). At the government pheasant breeding establishments in Thailand, faeces are removed within 24 hours, and this appears to have almost eliminated the transmission of coccidia; only a few oocysts were seen in four of the pheasants examined. Coccidia are generally host specific, and cross-infection to Green Peafowl is not likely to occur.

Cross-infection with helminth parasites does occur readily between different species of gallinaceous birds, but the level of worm infection in all the birds examined in Thailand appeared to be very low.

There are very few records of haematozoa from Asian peafowl (Bennett et al. 1982). The only species described is *Haemoproteus rileyi* from the Blue Peafowl in India (Malkani 1936). The illustrations and description are poor and lack any measurements. Although Malkani attributed the death of his peafowl to haemoproteid infection, the general non-pathogenicity of *Haemoproteus* spp. suggests that this claim should be viewed with some reservation as a concomitant infection with some other disease agent may have been the primary cause. The haemoproteid found in the present study is therefore tentatively identified as *H. rileyi*, a species which clearly requires redescription and further study as to its possible pathogenicity. The general absence of haematozoa in the captive birds was probably due to regular application of insecticide, which would have controlled potential vectors.

In captive Green Peafowl, the significance of the Rickettsia-like organism, similar to that described from other birds (Peirce 1972), is not known. Ticks were found only on the wild peafowl, and no rickettsiae were seen in the blood of the single wild bird examined. The vector and aetiology of this organism therefore, for the present, remain unknown.

On the present evidence, parasitic infections do not appear to pose problems for the existing wild population of Green Peafowl in Thailand, or for those in captivity in breeding stations. However, the sample examined was small and largely from adult birds. Further study and monitoring are required to establish the species of coccidial and helminth parasites present and their significance in juveniles. Further blood samples are required to determine whether *H. rileyi* or other haematozoan parasites play any significant role in Green Peafowl ecology.

ACKNOWLEDGEMENTS

We are grateful to Nopparat Naksatit, Theerapat Prayurasiddhi and Prateep Rojanadilok for their help at Huai Kha Kheng. Robert Atkinson, Nichola Gwynne-Howell and Rupert Quinnell assisted in collecting samples.

REFERENCES

BEJSOVEC, J. 1972. Coccidiosis in the pheasant *Phasianus colchicus* and in the partridge *Perdix perdix* in an agricultural area of Czechoslovakia. *J. Protozool.* **19** (Suppl) 75.
BEJSOVEC, J. 1977A. Persistence of coccidia in changing landscape with decreasing number of host animals. *J. Protozool.* **24** (4): 48A.
BEJSOVEC, J. 1977B. Seasonal fluctuation in the occurrence of the coccidian *Eimeria tetricis*, a parasite of black grouse. *J. Protozool.* **24** (2): 13A.
BEJSOVEC, J. 1978. Okologische einflusse auf die verbreitungsdynamik der kokzidienarten *Eimeria phasiani* und *Eimeria colchici*. *Angew. parasit.* **19**: 76–85.
BEJSOVEC, J. 1979. Coccidians in relic populations of the Capercaillie, *Tetrao urogallus*. *J. Protozool.* **26** (3): 39A.
BENNETT, G. F., WHITEWAY, M. & WOODWORTH-LYNAS, C. 1982. A host-parasite catalogue of the avian haematozoa. *Memorial Univ. Nfld. Occas. Pap. Biol.* No 5.
BHATIA, B. B. & PANDE, B. P. 1966. A new coccidium, *Eimeria mayurai* (Sporozoa: Eimeriidae) from the common peafowl *Pavo cristatus* L. *Proc. Nat. Acad. Sci. Ind.* Series B **36**: 39–42.
CARPENTER, J. W., SPRAKER, T. R. & NOVILLA, M. N. 1980. Disseminated visceral coccidiosis in Whooping Cranes. *J. Am. Vet. Med. Ass.* **177**: 845–8.
HILLGARTH, N. & STEWART COX, B. 1986. The decline of the Green Peafowl *Pavo muticus*. *Third International Pheasant Symposium*. Chang Mai, Thailand.
MAFF. 1977. *Manual of Veterinary Parasitological Laboratory Techniques*. Technical Bulletin No 18. HMSO. London.

MALKANI, P. G. 1936. *Haemoproteus rileyi* (sp. nov.) causing a fatal disease in Indian peacock. *Ind. J. Vet. Sci. Anim. Husb.* **6**: 155–7.
PATNAIK, M. M. 1966. Remarks on coccidia species from Indian peacock (*Pavo cristatus*). *Ind. J. Microbiol.* **6**: 53–4.
PEIRCE, M. A. 1972. Rickettsia-like organisms in the blood of *Turdus abyssinicus* in Kenya. *J. Wildl. Dis* **8**: 273–4.
PEIRCE, M. A. & PRINCE, P. A. 1980. *Hepatozoon albatrossi* sp. nov. (Eucoccidia: Hepatozoidae) from *Diomedea* spp. in the Antarctic. *J. Nat. Hist.* **14**: 447–52.
PELLÉRDY, L. 1974. *Coccidia and Coccidiosis* 2nd edition. Paul Parey, Berlin and Hamburg.

FAECAL BACTERIA IN UNHATCHED EGGS OF BOX-NESTING KESTRELS (*FALCO SPARVERIUS*)

PHOEBE BARNARD

*Hawk Mountain Sanctuary Association, Kempton, Pennsylvania, 19529
U.S.A., and
Department of Biology, Acadia University, Nova Scotia, B0P 1X0 Canada*

ABSTRACT

Eggs of the American Kestrel (*Falco sparverius*) were examined bacteriologically. Heavy growths of organisms were obtained. It is suggested that bacterial contamination associated with the use of nest-boxes may contribute to a reduction in egg hatchability. The American Kestrel is a useful model for the study of this and other factors.

INTRODUCTION

The American Kestrel (*Falco sparverius*) is not a threatened species; indeed, in some areas populations are expanding with both the clearing of land for small-scale agriculture, and the provision of artificial nest-boxes (Nagy 1963). However, the species represents a useful model for comparison with threatened species, particularly those nesting in cavities, and so I briefly describe here a qualitative bacteriological sample of eggs from a 'healthy' population. These results were initially printed in the Abstracts Manual of the 1982 Raptor Research Foundation Annual Meeting, but were not published in its Proceedings.

MATERIALS AND METHODS

Ten fully-incubated, intact, unhatched eggs from five kestrel nests were analysed. The nests were in untreated wooden boxes in mixed croplands, or in grazed or abandoned pastures, near narrow woodlots in eastern Pennsylvania, part of a large programme of next-box placement begun by the Hawk Mountain Sanctuary Association in the mid-1950s. Eggs were collected four to six days after the predicted hatch date, placed immediately in new zipper-sealing plastic bags, and frozen within two hours. Five to seven weeks later, the eggs were thawed for six hours at 22°C and carefully swabbed with 100 percent ethanol. Bacterial cultures were plated on standard nutrient agar using undiluted smears from both the emulsified egg contents and the inside of the shell membrane. Plates were streaked in duplicate and cultured for 24 hours at 37°C, and stored for up to 72 hours longer at 3°C; isolation plates were prepared if necessary after the first 24 hours. For possible future use, approximately 15ml of excess emulsion from each egg was cultured for 72 hours at 37°C in trypticase soy broth tubes. Standard physiochemical tests included the Gram stain, lactose-phenol red fermentation, urease production, Kligler's iron test for hydrogen sulphide, and routine examination for morphology and motility. Anaerobic techniques were not used. Bacteria were identified with the help of a laboratory manual provided by Dr F. Muzzopappa, and the identifications were subsequently confirmed by him. For more information, Cooper (1987) provides a thorough review of aerobic bacteriological and other techniques for raptor pathology studies (see also Scullion, this volume).

RESULTS

All ten eggs yielded large numbers of intestinal bacteria. Qualitatively, growths of *Streptococcus faecalis* and *Proteus vulgaris* were much more extensive than the limited growth of *Escherichia coli* (see also Needham 1981). One egg contained a well-differentiated embryo of about six to eight days, while the other nine were either infertile or had been killed before detectable differentiation.

DISCUSSION

Reproductive success of this population as a whole was low, with only 41–45 percent of eggs resulting in fledged young in 1982, the year of analysis. Since the first nest-boxes were provided, nest success has decreased (Heintzelman & Nagy 1968; Barnard 1982) and egg loss, including addling, infertility and predation, has increased. In 1980–1982, addled/infertile eggs accounted for 3.4–13.8 percent of all eggs laid, and 14.3–25.0 percent of the total egg/chick loss (Barnard 1982).

Similarly, in the captive American Kestrel population at McGill University, Canada, Bird (1981) has noted markedly reduced hatchability since inception of the captive breeding programme, and has thoroughly analysed its possible causes. In that population, bacterial contamination was not thought to have a significant effect. Study of the captive kestrel colony at Patuxent Research Station, USA, however, led Porter & Wiemeyer (1970) to postulate that *Streptococcus faecalis* and *Proteus* spp. are introduced on to eggshells via parental faeces, and enter the egg with moisture. If so, heat and humidity should facilitate contamination by shell pore expansion and the entry of condensation. Needham (1981), by contrast, suggested that contamination occurred during the laying process. It would be imprudent to conclude that bacterial pathogens caused developmental failure of the nine undifferentiated eggs in this study, but had the eggs simply been infertile and metabolically inactive, they should have resisted microbial invasion.

S. faecalis, *P. vulgaris* and *E. coli* are all cryoduric (able to withstand prolonged winter freezing). The 19 active nest-boxes in the study area in 1982 varied in the amount of fouling by excreta (*Figures 1* and *2*), which potentially poses a hazard to future clutches. Nelson (1971) suggested that wooden next-box walls may harbour bacteria during the winter; cryoduric organisms may survive in the untreated wood. There are, unfortunately, few data on egg hatchability in natural cavity-nesting birds, but nests protected from the weather, especially from direct sun, can be expected to harbour large ectoparasite populations (Olendorff & Stoddart 1974) and, logically, bacterial pathogens.

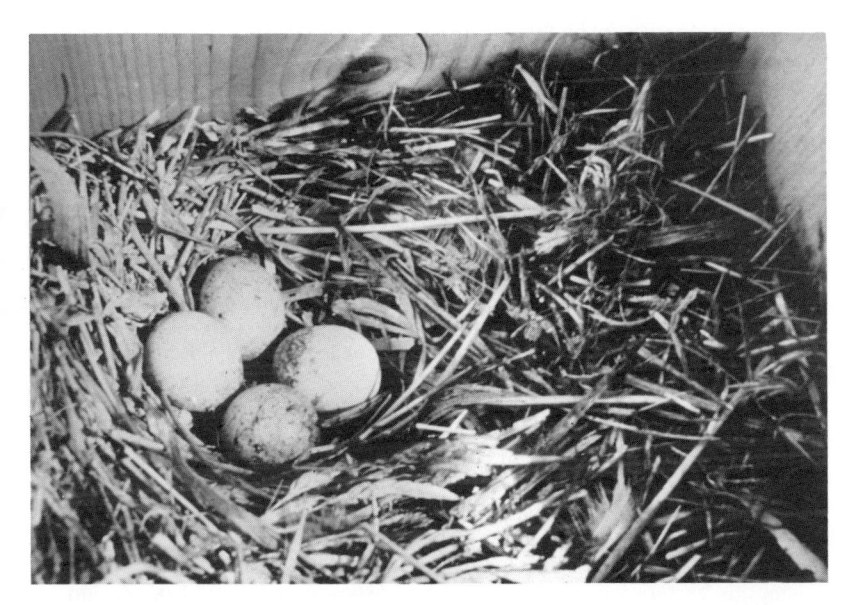

Figure 1: Clean nest-box of American Kestrel (*Falco sparverius*) in eastern Pennsylvania. (*Photo*: Jeanne Tinsman)

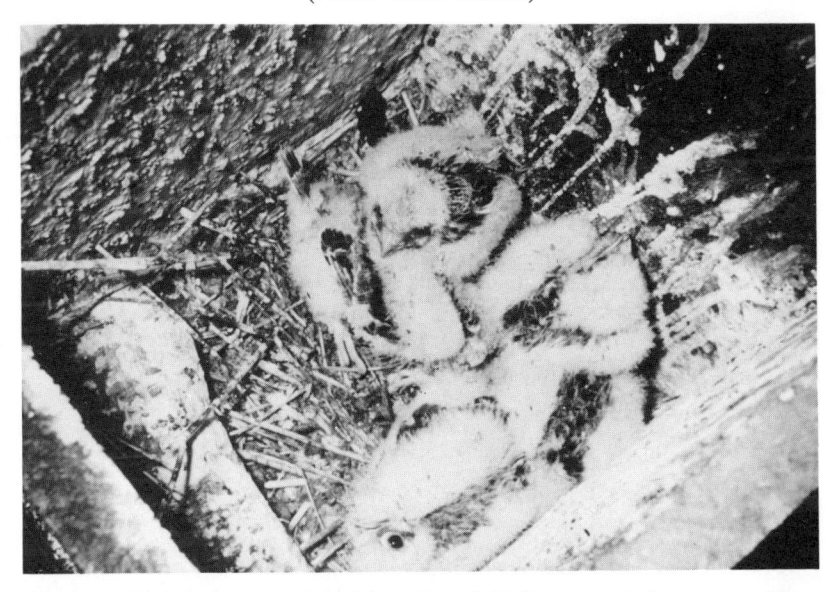

Figure 2: Fouled nest-box of American Kestrel (*Falco sparverius*) in eastern Pennsylvania. (*Photo*: Jeanne Tinsman)

Heintzelman (1971) speculated that nest-box sanitation in this kestrel population was not an important factor limiting egg hatchability. He observed three boxes in two sites, over seven different breeding seasons, with presumably different parents (potentially obscuring any relation between fouling and nest success), and he did not carry out bacteriological tests to substantiate his conclusions. Yet based on the observed hatchability rates of 86–97 percent (excluding predation), it is unlikely that nest-box sanitation does pose a major threat to this population. In addition to the population's expansion through the provision of artificial nest-sites, the species as a whole is resilient under ecological stress because of its large clutch size and early sexual maturity. However, this may not be true of some threatened cavity-nesting raptors, such as the Mauritius Kestrel (*Falco punctatus*) and some small owls, and researchers should include egg hatchability and nest fouling in their studies of threatened populations. In addition to possible pathological effects on adults (Needham *et al.* 1979; Cooper *et al.* 1981, 1986), bacteria may contaminate eggs or infect chicks in the closed environment of a nest cavity, especially under the intensive conditions of captive-breeding programmes.

ACKNOWLEDGEMENTS

I thank the staff of Hawk Mountain Sanctuary, particularly Jim Brett and Seth Benz, for their generous help and provision of breeding data from previous years; Frank Muzzopappa (Kutztown State College, Pennsylvania) for graciously placing his bacteriology laboratory at my disposal; and J. E. Cooper and an anonymous referee for constructive comments on the text.

FOOTNOTE

Author's present address: Department of Zoology, University of the Witwatersrand, Johannesburg 2050, Republic of South Africa.

REFERENCES

BARNARD, P. E. 1982. Breeding success and failure of the American Kestrel *Falco sparverius* in Berks and Lehigh Counties, Pennsylvania. Unpublished final report, Hawk Mountain Sanctuary Association Library, Kempton, PA, USA.

BIRD, D. M. 1981. Some microbial aspects of egg hatchability in captive American Kestrels. *In:* Cooper, J. E. & Greenwood, A. G. (eds). *Recent Advances in the Study of Raptor Diseases.* Chiron Publications, Keighley.

COOPER, J. E. 1987. Pathology. *In:* Pendleton, B. A. G., Millsap, B. A., Cline, K. W. & Bird, D. M. (eds). *Raptor Management Techniques Manual.* Institute for Wildlife Research, National Wildlife Federation Scientific and Technical Series No. 10, Washington D.C.

COOPER, J. E., JONES, C. G. & OWADALLY, A. W. 1981. Morbidity and mortality in the Mauritius Kestrel (*Falco punctatus*). *In:* Cooper, J. E. & Greenwood, A. G. (eds). *Recent Advances in the Study of Raptor Diseases.* Chiron Publications, Keighley.

COOPER, J. E., NEEDHAM, J. R. & FOX, N. C. 1986. Bacteriological, haematological and clinical chemical studies on the Mauritius Kestrel (*Falco punctatus*). *Avian Path.* **15**: 349–56.

HEINTZELMAN, D. S. 1971. Observations on the role of nestbox sanitation in affecting egg hatchability of wild Sparrow Hawks in eastern Pennsylvania. *Raptor Research News* **5**: 100–3.

HEINTZELMAN, D. S. & NAGY, A. C. 1968. Clutch sizes, hatchability rates, and sex ratios of Sparrow Hawks in eastern Pennsylvania. *Wilson Bull.* **80**: 306–11.

NAGY, A. C. 1963. Population density of Sparrow Hawks in eastern Pennsylvania. *Wilson Bull.* **75**: 93.

NEEDHAM, J. R. 1981. Bacterial flora of birds of prey. *In:* Cooper, J. E. & Greenwood, A. G. (eds). *Recent Advances in the Study of Raptor Diseases.* Chiron Publications, Keighley.

NEEDHAM, J. R., KIRKWOOD, J. K. & COOPER, J. E. 1979. A survey of the aerobic bacteria in the droppings of captive birds of prey. *Res. Vet. Sci.* **27**: 125–6.

NELSON, R. W. 1971. Captive breeding of Peregrines: suggestions from their behavior in the wild. *Raptor Research News* **5**: 54–82.

OLENDORFF, R. R. & STODDART, J. W. 1974. The potential for management of raptor populations in western grasslands. *Raptor Research Foundation Report* **2**: 47–87.

PORTER, R. D. & WIEMEYER, S. N. 1970. Propagation of captive American Kestrels. *J. Wildl. Manage.* **34**: 594–604.

LEGAL CONSIDERATIONS IN THE MOVEMENT AND SUBMISSION OF AVIAN SPECIMENS

MARGARET E. COOPER

35–43 Lincoln's Inn Fields, London WC2A 3PN, England

Note: This paper was given in outline at the Symposium on Disease and Management of Threatened Populations, and in greater detail together with *Table 1* at the XXIII World Veterinary Congress 1987, and the copyright of J. E. Cooper and M. E. Cooper in the table is acknowledged.

ABSTRACT

The problems of moving avian specimens from one country to another are outlined. Both disease and conservation controls must receive due consideration.

INTRODUCTION

There is an increasing interest in the role of disease and pathology in wild (free-living) populations because of the need to conserve rare or endangered species. Consequently, a number of conservation projects (and this is only restricted to avian populations for the purposes of this paper), often in remote parts of the world, are becoming involved in disease studies. In such places there may be particular difficulties of transportation, communications and environment (Omojola & Hanson 1986), and because of the need for specialized laboratory services it is often necessary to send samples, eggs or live birds out of the country in which they were taken, for study elsewhere. Furthermore, recent developments in the use of frozen bird semen promise to be a great asset in the rescue of declining populations by reducing the need to transport live birds in order to breed from them. However, legal controls apply to the movement of frozen semen when it is sent to different parts of the world, although a report in *The Times* on this subject suggests that there is a lack of awareness that controls apply to semen as well as to live birds (Morgan 1987).

If animals or animal material are to be sent across national boundaries, special consideration must be given to the legislative controls that are imposed in the course of exportation from the country of origin and importation into the country of destination. There are two separate fields of law involved, one providing protection against the spread of animal disease and the other restricting the trade in, and movement of, endangered species.

These restrictions are overlooked from time to time, for example when an important sample is posted to an overseas colleague or diagnostic laboratory without proper authorization. More often than not it arrives safely, but risks have been taken and almost invariably offences have been committed. To illustrate the risk: a British veterinary surgeon once received a fresh dog's head in the mail from overseas; it was very poorly wrapped and had been sent for rabies diagnosis in Great Britain, contrary to the strict import controls that are designed to keep this dangerous zoonosis out of the country. In many parts of the world there is close contact between domestic poultry and wild birds permitting the transmission of parasites or diseases which, if transported in infected material or live birds to another country, might endanger valuable national poultry flocks.

The penalties for violation of the importation laws of many countries include fines and/or imprisonment following a conviction. In addition, the material may be confiscated, destroyed or re-exported. Furthermore, the receiving person is put in a most difficult position since receipt puts them in possession of an illegally imported specimen. If this is rare and valuable material, does she/he report the matter and risk being told to destroy or surrender the specimen, or does she/he move deeper into illegality by processing the material, and perhaps thereby providing information which may be lifesaving or species-saving for the birds from which the samples were sent? Can the results be published if the illegality were thereby revealed? Clearly the only legal advice that can be offered is to declare the material immediately to the relevant authority and follow its instructions.

These problems can be avoided by following the required procedures. These will be outlined in general terms, showing the principles of animal health and endangered species controls which are likely to be encountered in most countries. A detailed table of the British law is provided at the end of this paper (*Table 1*) to show how such legislation works in practice. The regulations are altered frequently since it is necessary for the authorities to keep up to date with changes in disease patterns and in the classification of endangered species.

It is important, therefore, prior to each fresh importation procedure, to obtain the latest requirements and documentation from the country of destination. These should normally be available from the relevant government department either by direct application or through the embassy or high commission in the country of origin.

IMPORTATION

Two bodies of law must be considered when dealing with the importation of birds, particularly non-domesticated species:
 a) disease controls
 b) conservation controls.

These are normally administered by different government departments and will require separate applications and permits. An unfortunate illustration of this situation concerns a person who, just before returning to Britain, was given a parrot. He dutifully obtained all the disease control authorization that he required, but he did not realize that the parrot was also protected by British conservation laws governing importation and exportation of endangered species, and failed to obtain the necessary permits; consequently, his bird was confiscated on arrival and eventually repatriated to its country of origin.

a) Disease controls

The animal health legislation relating to bird imports is imposed in order to ensure that disease that may affect domestic avian species, including poultry, is not brought into the country. Permits to import have to be obtained in advance of arrival, from the destination country's government department responsible for agriculture. For example, in Britain the Ministry of Agriculture, Fisheries and Food, and in the United States (US) the Animal, Plant and Health Inspection Service of the US Department of Agriculture, deal with the requirements for these respective countries.

Conditions are imposed in such permits requiring, for example, that tests be carried out on live birds and that official veterinary certificates be obtained confirming the freedom, from specified diseases such as Newcastle disease, salmonellosis or egg drop syndrome, of the birds to be imported, of the flock from which they came, or of the country generally. Live specimens are normally subject to quarantine or isolation under veterinary supervision. In the case of dead birds and specimens, stipulations as to the use of transport or preservation medium (e.g. glutaraldehyde) or for the disposal of samples (e.g. by incineration on completion of tests) may be made; untreated samples may simply not be permitted. The particular requirements will vary according to the type, specimen, species, country of origin, destination and purpose for which the material is required.

b) Conservation controls

The Convention on International Trade in Endangered Species of Wild Fauna and Flora (otherwise known as the Washington Convention or CITES) has been signed and ratified by some 90 countries which have made the requirements of the Convention part of their legislation. The Convention provides a system which regulates the international movement, for trade and other purposes, of the non-domesticated species that are under various degrees of threat to their survival and which are consequently listed in Appendices I and II to the Convention.

The Convention not only applies to live birds but also to dead specimens, and, it is important to note, 'derivatives' of listed species. The term 'derivative' is defined in Article I of the Convention as any part which is readily recognizable as a part or derivative of a listed species. The European Community (EC) implementation of CITES by Council Regulation No. 3626/82 (as amended) refers to 'any other goods which appear from an accompanying document, the packaging or a mark or label, or from any other circumstances, to be parts or derivatives . . . unless specifically exempted . . .'. Recognition may, therefore, be by scientific analysis as well as visual identity and, as this definition is broad enough to include, for example, diagnostic samples taken from CITES-listed species, their importation into the EC requires a permit.

The type of permit and purpose for which import is permitted in respect of live birds depend on the category in which they are listed; Appendix I (endangered), for which import is restricted to scientific and similar purposes, or Appendix II (vulnerable), for which commercial trading permits may be available depending upon the species' conservation status. Some countries may apply Appendix I protection to certain Appendix II species; for example, the EC gives such treatment to all birds of prey. In addition, in Great Britain, even stricter controls apply which require documentation for any movement of birds of prey and their derivatives in or out of the country—despite the fact that there is normally free movement within the EC of species listed on CITES Appendices once such specimens have legally entered the EC via one member country. Species not listed in the CITES Appendices are not controlled, and therefore a permit is required only if there are other national restrictions in operation, although identification of 'free' species or their derivatives may be required by customs officials. There should be little problem obtaining permits of listed species for purposes such as scientific diagnosis; there are also specific exemptions for recognized institutions in respect of collected or exchanged material and specimens.

Import and export documentation is obtained from the CITES Management Authority in the relevant countries. In Britain this is the Department of the Environment, which also publishes guidance notes on the relevant controls (DOE 1987).

In Australia the Department of Primary Industries and Energy is preparing protocols for importation of certain exotic birds and hatching eggs (Wilson 1988).

The United States requirements are provided by Hoover (1984), and detailed information on endangered species controls can be obtained from the Office of Management Authority of the Department of the Interior, Fish and Wildlife Service. Permits under the Endangered Species Act and Migratory Bird Treaty Act may also be necessary (Garbe 1988).

EXPORTATION

Exportation is not normally a problem in respect of disease controls since a country is not generally concerned about what organisms or diseases are carried away from it, although difficulties can be encountered when a country does not wish, for political reasons, to advertise or have confirmed that a particular disease is present, especially if it may affect its export or tourist trade.

However, the conservation export controls are important since reciprocal documents generally have to be obtained from both the country of origin and of destination. Again, this may take time and diplomacy. Sometimes conditions are imposed, for example, on the exportation of a collection of specimens for a museum, a duplicate set of specimens or publications may have to be provided for the country of origin.

TRANSPORTATION

Any national or international requirements for the transportation of live birds or specimens (e.g. tissues, blood or faeces) must be observed. In the case of specimens, the import or export licence may specify a particular mode of packaging or transport. Postal regulations may restrict the kind of specimens that may be sent by mail: for example, in Britain there are special packaging instructions for the transmission of pathological specimens both nationally and internationally (Post Office, Annual; RCVS 1988). There are packing standards (IATA Annual) for live animals being transported by air which are enforced by most airlines and the CITES Secretariat has published guidance on the transportation of endangered species.

PRACTICAL PROBLEMS

On occasions, importation is entirely trouble-free; for instance when customs officers are well informed about or, conversely, are unaware of, the documentation that is required for an animal importation. On the other hand, importation can be traumatic, both for the importer and, when live animals are involved, for the imported creatures. Great delay can be caused, and live animals have been said to suffer, even die, while awaiting clearance for either import or export.

The sheer complexity may discourage or prevent scientists from supplying samples that have to be imported. Thus, a research worker wrote: 'I soon realized that sorting out any paperwork . . . was going to take up too much time. I therefore decided to concentrate on other aspects of my work'. In another field, a Mexican company had to decline to accept blood and feather samples from other countries because the delay in passing through customs formalities meant that samples, which required very prompt processing, were of no value.

On one occasion a rare pheasant made a double crossing of the Atlantic when essential health tests were omitted. The bird was rejected by the country of destination and had to return to its country of origin and wait in quarantine for the necessary tests and certification to be provided (Howman, undated).

The main problems of import and export include the following:

a) The time taken to obtain a permit. The bureaucratic processes involved in obtaining permits may lead to considerable delay, and applications should be submitted well in advance of the date when the import or export is intended to take place. Alternatively, arrangements should be made for the issue of permits at short notice. It may be necessary to allow time to clarify ambiguities or to obtain an official translation of documentation sent by the destination country. International postal services are often themselves subject to delay, and it may be necessary to use telex or facsimile as a faster, though more expensive, means of communication to get a satisfactory service.

b) The specimens involved. These must be clearly and precisely identified in the application for a permit. One of the problems when carrying out research in two separate countries is that one often cannot predict what specimens (in number or species) will be collected in the course of the project. Where the receiving country is helpful it is possible to make outline arrangements in advance (e.g. before departing on an expedition or visit to a project) and then to finalize the permit by telephone, facsimile or cable and arrange for the permits to be at the destination airport in time for the importer's arrival.

c) The terms of the licence. These may dictate how specimens are taken, packed, preserved, disinfected, tested for disease and finally stored or destroyed. It may be necessary to negotiate requirements which do not defeat a particular purpose or method of study.

d) Timing. Care must be taken that the licence or health certificates have not expired before the specimens are imported, and that any other dates on the documentation also match.

e) Charges. Import duty may be demanded, particularly in respect of live birds, even if they are imported for scientific purposes. Airport charges and the cost of employing a clearance agent may also have to be covered, in addition to postal or freight costs.

f) Documentation. Anyone who has dealt with import or export documentation will speak of the need to ensure that the wording of the paperwork is perfect,

Table 1: Diagnostic screening specimens from overseas—British requirements

Specimen	Preservation	MAFF Orders Poultry (see definitions)	MAFF Orders Other species	Application	DOE
Live birds		Yes 1, 2	Yes 1, 2	Order 1: all live birds	Live birds, carcasses, eggs (live or blown), plumage and any derivatives require import export permits if they are of species listed on EC Regulation 3626/82 as amended or if Endangered Species (Import and Export) Act 1976 (as amended) applies.
Carcasses	Fresh	Yes 2, 3	Yes 2	Order 2: only if material may be an animal pathogen or carrier thereof (see Definitions and Note 6)	
Carcasses	Fixed (e.g. in formalin or alcohol)	Yes* 3	No*	Order 3: products of poultry species B, C	Excepted species—no permit necessary but identification may be required by Customs officers.
				Order 4: species B	
Feathers	Fresh	Yes 2	Yes 2	Fixed material: Order 2 applies if it may be pathogenic	OGL for certain scientific institutions. See DOE Notice and Supplementary Notice No. 3.
Feathers	Fixed	No*	No*	*MAFF consider all material potentially to be subject to Order 2	Always check status with DOE or appropriate overseas authority. See DOE *Notice to Importers and Exporters* and *Supplementary Notices Nos. 1–6*.
Tissues	Fresh	Yes 2, 3	Yes 2		
Tissues	Fixed	Yes* 3	No*		
Parasites	Fresh	Yes 2	Yes 2		
Parasites	Fixed	Yes* 3	No*		

		MAFF	DOE
Faeces	Fresh	Yes 2, 3	Yes 2
Faeces	Fixed	Yes* 3	No*
Blood	In anticoagulant or serum	Yes 2, 3	Yes 2
Blood	Smears fixed	Yes* 3	No*
Eggs	Live for hatching	Yes 1, 2, 3	Yes 1, 2
Eggs	Fresh (not live)	Yes 2, 3	Yes 2
Eggs	Fixed	Yes* 3	No*
Semen	Fresh	Yes 2, 4	Yes* 4
Semen	Fixed	Yes* 4	Yes* 4

NOTES

1. Permits must be obtained prior to importation
2. Permits may be subject to conditions
   e.g. MAFF live birds—quarantine and health certificates specimens—disposal procedures
   e.g. DOE restriction for very rare species on place of keeping and on trade
3. There may be general licences operating in certain cases
4. CITES: export permits may be required

MAFF

LEGISLATION
1. Importation of Birds, Poultry and Hatching Eggs Order 1979 (A)
2. Importation of Animal Pathogens Order 1980 (B)
3. Importation of Animal Products and Poultry Products Order 1980 (as amended) (B, C)
4. Importation of Embryos, Ova and Semen Order 1980 (B)

DOE

LEGISLATION
EC Regulation EC 3626/82 as amended Endangered Species (Import and Export Act) 1976 as amended implementing CITES

DEFINITIONS
DERIVATIVES
any goods which appear from any accompanying document, the packaging or a mark or label, or from any other circumstances, to be parts or derivatives

Table 1—*continued*

5. EC: Member states generally accept CITES documentation issued by each other. However, stricter controls may exist
   e.g. UK import and export permits are required for eggs, plumage and diurnal birds of prey
6. MAFF: Fixed material is exempt from Order 2 only if it is not pathogenic. Consult MAFF prior to importation
7. MAFF/DOE requirements and the law change from time to time. The user of this summary is responsible for ascertaining the current position

DEFINITIONS
POULTRY:
A. live birds of every species
B. domestic fowls, turkeys, geese, ducks, guinea-fowls, pigeons, pheasants, partridges and quails
C. also grouse, ostriches, snipe, woodcock

ANIMAL PATHOGEN
any collection or culture or organisms which may cause disease in animals or poultry; or any animal material which may carry or transmit an animal pathogen (B)

ANIMAL PRODUCT
anything originating from live or dead poultry (B, C)
Includes: carcasses
Excludes: feathers, semen

ABBREVIATION
MAFF Ministry of Agriculture, Fisheries and Food

ADDRESS
Ministry of Agriculture, Fisheries and Food,
Hook Rise South,
Tolworth,
Surbiton,
Surrey KT6 7NF.
Tel. 01-336 4411

EXCEPTED SPECIES
Very common birds and derivatives as listed including domesticated species

BUT all plumage and live/blown eggs require a permit except for domesticated spp. as listed or per OGL, e.g. domestic fowls, turkeys, geese, ducks, pigeons. See DOE Notice

ABBREVIATIONS
DOE   Department of the Environment
CITES Convention on International Trade in Endangered Species of Wild Fauna and Flora (Washington Convention)
OGL   open general licence

ADDRESS
Department of the Environment,
Trade in Endangered Species Branch,
Tollgate House,
Houlton Street,
Bristol BS2 9DL.
Tel. 0272-218202

JOHN E. COOPER FRCVS
MARGARET E. COOPER LLB

precisely identifiable with the material or animals involved, and synchronized with the transport arrangements. Errors and omissions can be caused by authorities or owner or shipper, and Harris (1988) has listed some of the problems involved.

CONCLUSIONS

The importation and exportation of diagnostic specimens for the investigation of avian disease require a thorough understanding of the legal controls on the movement of such material. The requirements are important safeguards to restrict the spread of disease and to protect endangered species. Although they cause difficulty to scientists who pursue their studies in more than one country, nevertheless many birds and scientific specimens have been transported around the world successfully to the benefit of conservation, science and medicine.

REFERENCES

CITES 1980. *Guidelines for Transport and Preparation for Shipment of Live Animals and Plants.* Secretariat of the Convention on International Trade in Endangered Species of Wild Fauna and Flora, Gland.

DOE 1987. *Controls on the Import and Export of Endangered and Vulnerable Species, with supplementary notices 1–6.* Department of the Environment, Bristol.

GARBE, J. A. L. 1988. Wildlife Law. *In:* Wilson, J. F. (ed.). *Law and Ethics of the Veterinary Profession.* Priority Press, Yardley.

HARRIS, T. C. 1988. Incorrect veterinary certification. *Vet. Rec.* **122**: 143.

HOOVER, D. E. 1984. Basic regulations to know before importing birds. *Bird World* September 1984: 60–4.

HOWMAN, K. C. R. undated. *WPA Notes and News.* World Pheasant Association.

IATA Annual. *Live Animals Regulations.* International Air Transport Association, Geneva.

MORGAN, A. 1987. Frozen semen success in saving bird species. *The Times,* 14 August 1987.

OMOJOLA, E. & HANSON, R. P. 1986. Collection of diagnostic specimens from animals in remote areas. *World Animal Review* **60**: 38–40.

POST OFFICE Annual. *Post Office Guide.* Post Office, London.

RCVS 1988. *Dispatch of Pathological Specimens by Post.* Royal College of Veterinary Surgeons, London.

WILSON, D. 1988. Importation of live birds and hatching eggs. *Dander* (Newsletter of the Australian Veterinary Poultry Association) **31**: 2.

FURTHER READING

COOPER, M. E. 1987. *An Introduction to Animal Law.* Academic Press, London.

RCVS 1987. *Legislation Affecting the Veterinary Profession in the United Kingdom.* Royal College of Veterinary Surgeons, London.

WILSON, J. F. 1988. *Law and Ethics of the Veterinary Profession.* Priority Press, Yardley.

USEFUL ADDRESSES

Australia: Department of Primary Industries and Energy, GPO Box 858, Canberra, ACT 2601.

Great Britain: see *Table 1*

USA: Office of Management Authority, U.S. Fish and Wildlife Service, PO Box 27329, Central Station, Washington, DC 20038-7329.

Import-Export Operations Staff, Veterinary Services, APHIS USDA, Federal Building, 6505 Belcrest Road, Hyattsville, MD 20782.

CONCLUSIONS

J. E. COOPER

Royal College of Surgeons of England, 35–43 Lincoln's Inn Fields, London WC2A 3PN, England.

This volume has, of necessity, covered a wide range of topics. The opening papers by Rod Reece, Bruce Hunter, Gwyn Ashton and Francis Scullion provide background information on pathogens and these papers are primarily intended to assist ornithologists, ecologists and field workers who, while often specialists in their own field, are usually relatively unfamiliar with micro-organisms and parasites. Succeeding papers discuss the possible role of pathogens in threatened populations, in some cases predominantly in theoretical terms, in others based on studies in the field. John Cooper outlines the history of the topic and draws attention to the fact that only relatively recently have infectious and parasitic diseases been seriously considered in studies on rare or localized species. Steven McOrist's paper is a post-mortem survey of birds that are not yet classified as 'threatened', but the work is important because 1) Australia is relatively isolated, partly on account of its geographical location but also because of the strict legal controls on birds entering and leaving the country, 2) there was little previous work on causes of mortality in the species in question, and 3) the findings show the value of surveys of diseases of free-living birds. The incidence of psittacine beak and feather disease, in particular, is a timely reminder of the threat presented by some pathogens to threatened populations, and reiterates the much repeated point that national monitoring centres are necessary if wildlife disease is to be studied and evaluated.

Michael Peirce discusses haematozoa and points out that while wild birds do not generally succumb to these parasites they may do so if suffering from intercurrent disease or if exposed for the first time because of the introduction of the parasite or its vector. David Jenkins and his colleagues provide convincing evidence for the role of exotic diseases, especially avian malaria and pox, in the decline of the endangered Hawaiian Crow. Only a small part appeared to be played by infectious disease in mortality of captive Pink Pigeons studied by Carl Jones and colleagues, but their paper illustrates very well the need to analyse causes of ill-health and death in all captive breeding programmes for threatened species and, where possible, for similar research to be performed in the field. On the other hand, James Carpenter and colleagues record a disastrous outbreak of a viral disease in captive Whooping Cranes: the case report illustrates the vulnerability of isolated populations, both in captivity and free-living, to certain infectious agents. Bill Bourne's paper emphasizes the threat not only to wild birds but also to domestic animals and even humans of the spread of pathogens. The work of Nigella Hillgarth and colleagues on the Green Peafowl demonstrate the value of monitoring parasites in threatened birds and the need to consider this an integral part of any management programme. Phoebe Barnard's paper deals with a species of bird that is certainly *not* threatened—the American Kestrel. However, her studies on faecal bacteria illustrate that this species—and, indeed, others—can be excellent models for studying the mechanisms of disease and infection which are of relevance to rarer birds.

It is clear from these Proceedings that more attention could and should be paid to the role of disease in threatened populations. This necessitates a fresh approach by avian research workers who must either become accomplished at screening and examining birds themselves—no easy task—or work more closely with veterinarians and others who can provide the necessary expertise. The latter—multidisciplinary—approach would appear to be the way forward and for this reason the appendices include a list of laboratories and reference centres and protocols for screening. Legal considerations are discussed in Margaret Cooper's paper: national controls on the movement of tissues and samples may appear irksome but must be observed if those working in this field are to retain their credibility with the appropriate authorities. The appendices will help those who need assistance in investigating outbreaks of disease or the examination of samples, or who require guidance in the taking and storage of diagnostic material.

At the end of the ICBP symposium in Kingston, the following two resolutions were put forward.

1. ICBP should note that there is increasing evidence that infectious and parasitic disease may have an adverse impact on avian populations and should encourage health monitoring in all studies on, and management programmes for, threatened species.

2. National and international bodies and governments should be made aware of the potential dangers to domestic stock and humans, as well as to wildlife, of the movement of birds and their products from one country to another. These groups should be urged to introduce controls so as to restrict the risk of spread of avian pathogens, especially to isolated populations.

The arguments for such measures remain as strong today as they did at the time of the symposium. All those concerned for the long-term survival of the world's avifauna should do their utmost to press for appropriate action. Ways in which this might be achieved are outlined in many papers in this book. In particular there is a need to increase awareness amongst conservationists and field biologists of the importance of monitoring disease. This can be done by publishing literature (such as this book), by organizing meetings, and by promoting both formal and informal links between biologists and veterinarians. The establishment of more reference collections of pathological material, on the lines of the Mascarene Collection in London (Cooper & Jones 1986), and international computer banks detailing the global distribution of pathogens, vectors and hosts, would help provide background data for those working in this field. In addition to all this, however, research is urgently needed, particularly the monitoring of free-living populations for infection/disease and studies (on both free-living and captive birds) on such factors as host susceptibility to pathogens, innate versus acquired immunity, and the feasibility of increasing the resistance of vulnerable species by (*inter alia*) vaccination and genetic selection.

ICBP is to be congratulated on its initiative in organizing this symposium and its courage in permitting papers on such a diverse range of subjects—in some cases reporting work that is still at an embryonic stage—to be put together as a

Technical Publication. There can be little doubt that this subject will assume increasing importance in years to come, as avian populations become more threatened, spread of pathogens is facilitated, and 'new' wildlife diseases are recognized. This volume will, we hope, prove to be an important landmark in ensuring that the interaction between birds and pathogenic organisms is fully appreciated. At the same time, it may help to emphasize that veterinarians, microbiologists, parasitologists and epidemiologists all have a part to play in studies on wild birds. This book is going to print at a time when ICBP has launched its new 'Biodiversity Project'. In his introduction to this the Director of ICBP stated:

> 'To preserve the world's biodiversity is a huge interdisciplinary task. . . . To render our work really useful for the international conservation community, a key element . . . is to consult closely with many other organisations and experts' (Imboden 1988).

It is to be hoped that by involving and attracting scientists from a variety of disciplines both the symposium in 1986 and these Proceedings will have made some contribution towards this aim.

REFERENCES

COOPER, J. E. & JONES, C. G. 1986. A reference collection of endangered specimens. *Linnean* 2: 32.

IMBODEN, C. 1986. The need for interdisciplinary co-operation. *World Birdwatch* 10(2): 2.

APPENDIX 1

REGISTER OF LABORATORIES AND REFERENCE CENTRES

Compiled by

N. Hillgarth[1] & J. E. Cooper[2]

1 *Department of Zoology, South Parks Road, Oxford OX1 3PS, England*
2 *Royal College of Surgeons of England, 35–43 Lincoln's Inn Fields, London WC2A 3PN, England*

INTRODUCTION

The aims of the Register are as follows:

1. To have a list of people to whom live or dead birds, or specimens from them, may be submitted.
2. To provide names of persons who may be consulted over problems relating to morbidity and mortality.
3. To facilitate exchange of information and material between those working on avian diseases.

The Register is divided into two parts; the first consists of a geographical list and index, the second comprises the submissions of those included on the Register. It should be noted that the latter are arranged in alphabetical order and that the style used follows that submitted by the registrant; thus, for example, some people have their first names listed while others are referred to only by initial.

Those sending live birds or pathological material from one country to another should be aware of the possible legal restrictions on movement and ensure that the relevant documentation is obtained (see M. E. Cooper, this volume).

We recognize that the Register is far from complete, but hope that it will go some way to fostering closer contact between those working on avian diseases and allow their work to be readily accessible to colleagues in other disciplines.

PART 1: GEOGRAPHICAL LIST

COUNTRY	NAME
AUSTRALIA	BARRETT, Kim
	BLACK, Douglas
	DINGLE, John G.
	FARAGHER, Trevor
	HARTLEY, W. J.
	HARRIGAN, Karl
	JONES, Hugh I.
	MACWHIRTER, Patricia
	MADILL, David
	MASON, R. W.
	McORIST, S.
	MOONEY, Nick
	OLSEN, Penny & Jerry
BRAZIL	DA SILVA, G. M.
CANADA	AYLARD, K. W.
	BENNETT, Gordon F.
	BIRD, David M.
	BISHOP, M.
	CAINES, J.
	CUSHMAN, Charlotte
	FALLIS, A. M.
	FITZGERALD, Guy
	INTERNATIONAL REFERENCE CENTRE FOR AVIAN HAEMATOZOA
	KEY, Douglas W.
CHILE	TORRES, Patricio H.
EAST GERMANY (GDR)	HENTSCHEL, Peter
FRANCE	CADOT, Pierre J.
	DEMEAUTIS, Georges
	GUIRAUD, Claude
NIGERIA	ADENE, Dan F.
NETHERLANDS	DORRESTEIN, Gerry M.
SPAIN	ARANDA, Francisco
	DEL CAMPO, A. L. Garcia
	STORM, Johanna
SOUTH AFRICA (RSA)	HUCHZERMEYER, F. W.
	KEMP, A.
	LEDGER, John
	INSTITUTE FOR MEDICAL RESEARCH
	VETERINARY RESEARCH INSTITUTE

Appendix 1: Register of Laboratories etc. 157

COUNTRY	NAME
SWEDEN	MORNER, Torsten
UNITED ARAB EMIRATES	McKINNEY, P.
	REMPLE, John D.
	RIDDLE, Kenton E.
UNITED KINGDOM	BEER, J. V.
	COOKE, Stephen
	COOPER, John E.
	GARNHAM, P. C. C.
	GREENWOOD, A. G.
	KEYMER, I. F.
	KIRKWOOD, James K.
	NEWTON, Ian
	PEIRCE, M. A.
	REECE, Rodney, L.
	SCULLION, Francis
UNITED STATES OF AMERICA	APANIUS, Victor
	ASSOCIATION OF AVIAN VETERINARIANS
	BUTCHER, Gary D.
	CONVERSE, Kathryn
	COSGROVE, Gerald E.
	CLARKE, Rick
	CLAYTON, Dale H.
	DEPARTMENT OF THE INTERIOR, FISH AND WILDLIFE SERVICE
	DEIN, F. Joshua
	FRANSON, J.
	FORRESTER, D. J.
	FOWLER, Murray E.
	FRIEND, Milton
	GOODWIN, Mark A.
	GRAHAM, David
	HARMON, Wallace M.
	HUNTER, David
	INTERNATIONAL WILDLIFE VETERINARY SERVICE
	JESSUP, David
	KOCK, Nancy
	KOCK, Mike
	LOCKE, Louis
	LOWENSTINE, Linda
	McALLISTER, Harold
	McNAMARA, Tracey
	McLEAN, Robert G.
	MIYASKI, Peggy
	NETTLE, Victor F.
	ODER, Edwin M.
	OUTLAW, Jennifer

COUNTRY	NAME
UNITED STATES OF AMERICA *continued*	PHILIPS, James R. POKRAS, Mark A. RHOADES, Keith R. ROERTEGEN, Karen ROFFE, Thomas SEGDWICK, Charles J. SILEO, Louis SOUCY, L. J. SPALDING, Marilyn THOMAS, Nancy TUFTS UNIVERSITY SCHOOL OF VETERINARY MEDICINE—WILDLIFE CLINIC WELLS, Susan WINDINGSTAD, Ron WILLIAMS, Elizabeth S.
WEST GERMANY (FRG)	BÖTTCHER, Martin KÖSTERS, Josef VOGT, Dagmar
YUGOSLAVIA	OSVEGY, Josef
VENEZUELA	GABALDON, Arnoldo

PART 2: LIST OF REGISTRANTS

NAME: ADDRESS:	ADENE, Dan F. DVM, MVSc Department of Veterinary Medicine Avian Medicine Section University of Ibadan NIGERIA
INTERESTS:	Avian medicine and pathology.
WILLING TO BE CONSULTED ON:	Related subjects.
WOULD WELCOME INFORMATION ON:	Management and disease control.
CAN PROVIDE INFORMATION ON:	Diagnosis and disease control.

Appendix 1: Register of Laboratories etc.

NAME:	APAINUS, Victor BSc
ADDRESS:	Department of Zoology
	University of Pennsylvania
	Philadelphia PA 1904-6018
	UNITED STATES OF AMERICA
INTERESTS:	Impact of haematozoa on wild populations, avian immunology, comparisons of immune parameters of wild and captive-reared birds.
WILLING TO BE CONSULTED ON:	Immunology.
WOULD WELCOME INFORMATION ON:	Serum or blood smears from birds with suspected immunological disorders.
CAN PROVIDE INFORMATION ON:	Analysis of immunoglobulin isotypes in serum or body fluids.

NAME:	ARANDA, Francisco A. LCB
ADDRESS:	Gran Via 48 2 Planta
	18010 Granada
	SPAIN
INTERESTS:	Conservation and rehabilitation of birds.
WILLING TO BE CONSULTED ON:	Clinical care, rehabilitation.
WOULD WELCOME INFORMATION ON:	Clinical care, pathological examination, diagnostic laboratory techniques, rehabilitation.

NAME:	AYLARD, K. W. BSA, DVM
ADDRESS:	Alberni Veterinary Clinic Ltd.
	Site 213 C-7 Nanaimo HWY
	Port Alberni B.C. V9Y 7L6
	CANADA
INTERESTS:	Clinical treatment, especially orthopaedics.
WILLING TO BE CONSULTED ON:	Clinical care.
WOULD WELCOME INFORMATION ON:	Clinical care, clinical pathology.

NAME:	BARRETT, Kim BVSc
ADDRESS:	Launceston Veterinary Clinic 351 Wellington Street Launceston TASMANIA AUSTRALIA 7249
INTERESTS:	Treatment and clinical care of injured and diseased wildlife.
WILLING TO BE CONSULTED ON:	Clinical care, rehabilitation, radiography.
WOULD WELCOME INFORMATION ON:	Physiotherapy techniques.
CAN PROVIDE INFORMATION ON:	Anaesthesia, surgical techniques.

NAME:	BEER, J. V. BSc, PhD, DipBact, CBiol, MIBiol
ADDRESS:	The Game Conservancy Fordingbridge Hants SP6 1EF UNITED KINGDOM
INTERESTS:	Avian pathology.
WILLING TO BE CONSULTED ON:	Pathological examination, diagnostic laboratory techniques, parasitology, rehabilitation, mycoses.
WOULD WELCOME INFORMATION ON:	Gamebird diseases.
CAN PROVIDE INFORMATION ON:	Gamebird, wildfowl and gull diseases.

NAME:	BENNETT, Gordon F. BA, MA, PhD
ADDRESS:	International Reference Centre for Avian Haematozoa Memorial University of Newfoundland St John's, Newfoundland CANADA
INTERESTS:	Avian haematozoa (blood parasites)—taxonomy, life-cycles, impact on wild populations.
WILLING TO BE CONSULTED ON:	Identification of parasites in blood smears, experimental procedures for studying blood parasites of birds, field techniques for obtaining birds, and vectors of blood parasites.

WOULD WELCOME INFORMATION ON:	Blood smears from wild or zoo populations anywhere in the world, reprints of articles on blood parasites of birds.
CAN PROVIDE INFORMATION ON:	Host-parasite catalogue and bibliographies of avian blood parasites, extensive reprint collection of the world's literature on blood parasites of birds—could provide a copy of specific papers. *See entry under International Reference Centre for Avian Haematozoa.*

NAME:	BIRD, David M. BSc, MSc, PhD
ADDRESS:	Macdonald Raptor Research Centre of McGill University 21, 111 Lakeshore Road Ste. Anne De Bellevue Quebec H9X 1C0 CANADA
INTERESTS:	All aspects of biology and management of birds of prey.
WILLING TO BE CONSULTED ON:	Clinical care, toxicology, rehabilitation, reproductive physiology.
WOULD WELCOME INFORMATION ON:	Open to all fields.
CAN PROVIDE INFORMATION ON:	Bird of prey management.

NAME:	BLACK, Douglas BVSc, MACVSc
ADDRESS:	570 Springvale Road Springvale South 3172 Victoria AUSTRALIA
INTERESTS:	Caged and aviary bird medicine and surgery.
WILLING TO BE CONSULTED ON:	Related subjects.

NAME:	BÖTTCHER, Martin DVM
ADDRESS:	PO Box 2164 5372 Schleiden WEST GERMANY
INTERESTS:	Avian medicine and pathology.
WILLING TO BE CONSULTED ON:	Related subjects and endoscopy.
WOULD WELCOME INFORMATION ON:	Trace elements in feathers.

NAME:	BUTCHER, Gary D. BS, DVM, PhD
ADDRESS:	Department of Preventive Medicine Box J-136, JHMHC, CVM Gainsville, FL 32611 UNITED STATES OF AMERICA
INTERESTS:	Poultry-layers, broilers, turkeys, pet birds, gamebirds.
WILLING TO BE CONSULTED ON:	Pathological examination, diagnostic laboratory techniques and parasitology.
CAN PROVIDE INFORMATION ON:	Avian diseases.

NAME:	CADOT, Pierre J. DVM
ADDRESS:	BP 16 14 rue Florian 28260 Anet FRANCE
INTERESTS:	Emergency wild animal medicine, dermatology.
WILLING TO BE CONSULTED ON:	Related subjects and orthopaedics.

NAME:	CLAYTON, Dale H. BA MS
ADDRESS:	Committee on Evolutionary Biology 1025 East 57 Street Chicago IL 60637 UNITED STATES OF AMERICA
INTERESTS:	Behavioural ecology of avian parasite interactions, Mallophaga systematics.

NAME:	COOKE, Stephen Warnes BVSc, MRCVS
ADDRESS:	Cygnus House 5 Beechwood Close Ascot Berkshire SL5 8QJ UNITED KINGDOM
INTERESTS:	Avian surgery and medicine, lead and tetra ethyl lead poisoning.
WILLING TO BE CONSULTED ON:	Related subjects, but not toxicology except lead poisoning.
CAN PROVIDE INFORMATION ON:	Related subjects.

Appendix 1: Register of Laboratories etc.

NAME:	COOPER, John E. BVSc, CertLAS, DTVM, MRCPath, FIBiol, FRCVS
ADDRESS:	Royal College of Surgeons of England Lincoln's Inn Fields London WC2A 3PN UNITED KINGDOM
INTERESTS:	Pathology, clinical diagnosis, laboratory techniques, health monitoring.
WILLING TO BE CONSULTED ON:	Related subjects.
CAN PROVIDE INFORMATION ON:	Clinical and post-mortem data, advice on pathological material.

NAME:	COSGROVE, Gerald E. MD
ADDRESS:	Zoological Society, San Diego PO Box 551 Pathology San Diego, CA 92112
OR	Silverwood Wildlife Sanctuary 13003 Wildeal Canyon Road Lakeside, CA 92040 UNITED STATES OF AMERICA
INTERESTS:	Pathology, parasitology.
WILLING TO BE CONSULTED ON:	Related subjects.
WOULD WELCOME INFORMATION ON:	Summaries or reprints of work.
CAN PROVIDE INFORMATION ON:	Work on bird diseases and parasites.

NAME:	CUSHMAN, Charlotte BA, DVM
ADDRESS:	3 Killarney Gardens Pointe Claire Quebec CANADA
INTERESTS:	Raptor medicine.
WILLING TO BE CONSULTED ON:	Related subjects.

NAME:	DA SILVA, G. M. Professor
ADDRESS:	Rua Vital Brazil Filito No. 64
	Niliror Cep 24.000
	Faculdade De Veterinaria Universidade Federal
	Fluminense, UFF
	BRAZIL
INTERESTS:	Diagnostic laboratory techniques.
WILLING TO BE CONSULTED ON:	Diagnostic laboratory techniques and parasitology.
WOULD WELCOME INFORMATION ON:	Pathology and parasitology.
CAN PROVIDE INFORMATION ON:	Immunology.

NAME:	DEIN, F. Joshua, VMD, MS
ADDRESS:	National Wildlife Research Center
	United States Fish and Wildlife Service
	6006 Schroeder Road
	Madison, WI 53711
	UNITED STATES OF AMERICA
INTERESTS:	Avian clinical pathology, care of wildlife as experimental animals.
WILLING TO BE CONSULTED ON:	Clinical care, rehabilitation.
CAN PROVIDE INFORMATION ON:	Assorted reprints and teaching materials.

NAME:	DEL CAMPO, Antonio Louis Garcia
	Veterinary Surgeon
ADDRESS:	Amparo Usera 25
	28026 Madrid
	SPAIN
INTERESTS:	Wild birds.
WILLING TO BE CONSULTED ON:	Clinical care, pathological examination, rehabilitation.

NAME:	DEMEAUTIS, Georges Veterinary Surgeon, DEA, Eco-Ethology
ADDRESS:	36 rue Baudrimont Toulouse FRANCE
INTERESTS:	Surgery, laboratory investigation and treatment in wild animals.
WILLING TO BE CONSULTED ON:	Related subjects, especially rehabilitation.
WOULD WELCOME INFORMATION ON:	Laboratory investigation and treatment in wild birds.
CAN PROVIDE INFORMATION ON:	Rehabilitation of wild birds (raptors).
NAME:	DINGLE, John G. BVSc, PhD, Grad Dip Ed, MRCVS, MACE, MAIAS
ADDRESS:	Queensland Agricultural College Lawes 4343 Queensland AUSTRALIA
INTERESTS:	Diseases of wild birds.
WILLING TO BE CONSULTED ON:	Clinical care, pathological examination, rehabilitation.
NAME:	DORRESTEIN, Gerry M. DVM, PhD
ADDRESS:	Department of Laboratory and Special Animal Diseases Faculty of Veterinary Medicine Yalelaan 1 3584 CL Utrecht THE NETHERLANDS
INTERESTS:	Avian pathology, avian pharmacotherapy, and kinetics.
WILLING TO BE CONSULTED ON:	Pathological examination, diagnostic laboratory techniques, parasitology, toxicology.
WOULD WELCOME INFORMATION ON:	Pharmacokinetic studies of drugs in birds.
CAN PROVIDE INFORMATION ON:	As above.

NAME:	FARAGHER Trevor PhD, BVSc, DipBact, MRCVS
ADDRESS:	National Biological Standards Laboratory Private Bag No 7 Parkville 3052 AUSTRALIA
INTERESTS:	Avian virology and vaccines.
WILLING TO BE CONSULTED ON:	Diagnostic laboratory techniques.

NAME:	FITZGERALD, Guy DMV
ADDRESS:	Faculty of Veterinary Medicine 3200 Sicotte, CP 5000 St Hyacinthe, Quebec J2S 7C6 CANADA
INTERESTS:	Raptor rehabilitation.
WILLING TO BE CONSULTED ON:	Related subjects and anaesthesia.
WOULD WELCOME INFORMATION ON:	Nutrition and calcium supplementation, data on reproduction.
CAN PROVIDE INFORMATION ON:	Avian anaesthesia.

NAME:	FOWLER, Murray E. DVM
ADDRESS:	University of California Davis School of Veterinary Medicine Department of Medicine Davis, California 95616 UNITED STATES OF AMERICA
INTERESTS:	Clinical medicine.
WILLING TO BE CONSULTED ON:	Related subjects.
CAN PROVIDE INFORMATION ON:	Experiences in clinical medicine.

Appendix 1: Register of Laboratories etc.

NAME:	FRIEND, Milton BS, MS, PhD
ADDRESS:	Director, National Wildlife Health Research Center 6006 Schroeder Road Madison, Wisconsin 53711 UNITED STATES OF AMERICA
INTERESTS:	Epizootiology, diseases of free-living wildlife, avian pathology, disease control, teaching, interactions between chemical and microbial agents, lead poisoning, avian diseases.
WILLING TO BE CONSULTED ON:	Pathological examination, diagnostic laboratory techniques, toxicology, disease control, training others in disease identification and control.
WOULD WELCOME INFORMATION ON:	Causes of mortality in free-living populations of endangered species, lead poisoning in wildlife, inclusion body disease of cranes, avian cholera, avian botulism, duck plague.
CAN PROVIDE INFORMATION ON:	As above.

NAME:	GOODWIN, Mark A. BS, DVM, MAM, PhD
ADDRESS:	PO Box 20 Oakwood Road Oakwood, GA 30566 UNITED STATES OF AMERICA
INTERESTS:	Diagnostic and experimental pathology.
WILLING TO BE CONSULTED ON:	Pathological examination, light microscopy and ultrastructure, and diagnostic laboratory techniques.
WOULD WELCOME INFORMATION ON:	Fixed specimens, histologic sections, references on new findings, rare diseases.
CAN PROVIDE INFORMATION ON:	As above.

NAME:	GRAHAM, David
ADDRESS:	Texas A&M University College Station Texas UNITED STATES OF AMERICA
INTERESTS:	Avian medicine and pathology.

NAME:	GREENWOOD, A. G. MA, VetMB, MRCVS, MIBiol
ADDRESS:	International Zoo Veterinary Group Hainsworth House Damems Lane Keighley West Yorkshire UNITED KINGDOM
INTERESTS:	Avian medicine and pathology.
WILLING TO BE CONSULTED ON:	Related subjects.

NAME:	GUIRAUD, Claude DVM
ADDRESS:	Route de Pau 65420 Ibos FRANCE
INTERESTS:	Raptors.
WILLING TO BE CONSULTED ON:	Clinical care and pathological examination.
WOULD WELCOME INFORMATION ON:	*Gyps fulvus*.

NAME:	HARMON, Wallace M. PhD
ADDRESS:	Department of Biology California State University Fresno, CA 93711 UNITED STATES OF AMERICA
INTERESTS:	Parasitology (avian haematozoa, *Trichomonas gallinae*, spiruroid infections of raptors).
WILLING TO BE CONSULTED ON:	Parasitology.
WOULD WELCOME INFORMATION ON:	Identification of microfilariae from birds.

Appendix 1: Register of Laboratories etc.

NAME:	HARRIGAN, Karl BVSc
ADDRESS:	University of Melbourne Veterinary Clinical Centre Werribee, Victoria AUSTRALIA 3030
INTERESTS:	Pathology/histopathology of avian disease, coccidiosis, pathological aspects of parasitism, penguin diseases.
WILLING TO BE CONSULTED ON:	Pathological examination, diagnostic laboratory techniques, parasitology but not taxonomy.
WOULD WELCOME INFORMATION ON:	Taxonomic identification of avian lice and identification of avian cestodes.
CAN PROVIDE INFORMATION ON:	Limited availability of histological sections of some diseases of wild birds.

NAME:	HARTLEY, W. J. FRCVS, FRCPath, MVSc, DSc
ADDRESS:	c/o Taronga Zoo, PO Box 20 Mosman, NSW 2088 AUSTRALIA
WILLING TO BE CONSULTED ON:	Pathological examination, diagnostic laboratory techniques, histopathology, parasitology, protozoology.
WOULD WELCOME INFORMATION ON:	Protozoan diseases.
CAN PROVIDE INFORMATION ON:	Comprehensive collection of materials relating to diseases of native fauna in SW Pacific area.

NAME:	HENTSCHEL, Peter DMV
ADDRESS:	Dabruner Str. 24 Pratau 4601 EAST GERMANY (GDR)
INTERESTS:	Diseases of birds of prey and owls.
WILLING TO BE CONSULTED ON:	Clinical care, diagnostic laboratory techniques, parasitology.
WOULD WELCOME INFORMATION ON:	Diseases of birds of prey including owls.
CAN PROVIDE INFORMATION ON:	Diseases of birds of prey including owls.

NAME:	INTERNATIONAL REFERENCE CENTRE FOR AVIAN HAEMATOZOA
ADDRESS:	Memorial University of Newfoundland St John's, Newfoundland CANADA
INTERESTS:	The Centre is the recognized repository for avian blood parasite material; and is willing to collaborate in studies on avian haematozoa with anyone.
MEMBERS:	BENNETT, G. F. Head (See separate entry) BISHOP, M. Research Assistant CAINES, J. Research Assistant WOODWORTH-LYNAS, C. Associate Research Curator
CORRESPONDING ASSOCIATES:	FALLIS, A. M. Professor Emeritus Department of Microbiology and Parasitology University of Toronto CANADA FORRESTER, D. J. College of Veterinary Medicine University of Florida UNITED STATES OF AMERICA GABALDON, Arnoldo Institute National de Higiene Caracas VENEZUELA GARNHAM, P. C. C. Professor Imperial College Ascot UNITED KINGDOM HUCHZERMEYER, F. W. Faculty of Veterinary Medicine University of Pretoria SOUTH AFRICA JONES, Hugh I. Department of Zoology University of Western Australia Nedlands, Western Australia AUSTRALIA PEIRCE, M. A. (see separate entry) 16 Westmorland Close Woosehill Wokingham, Berkshire UNITED KINGDOM

NAME:	INTERNATIONAL WILDLIFE VETERINARY SERVICE
ADDRESS:	PO Box 1413 Orangeville, CA 95662-1413 UNITED STATES OF AMERICA
INTERESTS:	Avian medicine and pathology.
MEMBERS:	CLARK, Rick HUNTER, David JESSUP, David KOCK, Nancy KOCK, Mike MIYASKI, Peggy

NAME:	JESSUP, David A. DVM, MPVM
ADDRESS:	PO Box 1413 International Wildlife Veterinary Service Orangevale, CA 95662 UNITED STATES OF AMERICA
INTERESTS:	Infectious diseases of free-flying birds.
WILLING TO BE CONSULTED ON:	Pathological examination, diagnostic laboratory techniques, waterfowl, marine and shorebird diseases, capture of wild birds.
WOULD WELCOME INFORMATION ON:	Toxicology and significant parasitology of wild birds.
CAN PROVIDE INFORMATION ON:	Waterfowl diseases, capture of wild birds.

NAME:	KEMP, A. PhD
ADDRESS:	Bird Department Transvaal Museum Box 413 Pretoria 0001 SOUTH AFRICA
CAN PROVIDE MATERIALS:	From the museum collections—alcohol and skeletal specimens.

NAME:	KEY, Douglas W. MSc, DVM
ADDRESS:	Ontario Ministry of Agriculture and Food Veterinary Services Laboratory PO Box 3612, Guelph, Ontario N1H 6R8 CANADA
INTERESTS:	Avian diagnostic virology—serology, virus isolation, development of diagnostic techniques including *Chlamydia*.
WILLING TO BE CONSULTED ON:	Diagnostic laboratory techniques.
WOULD WELCOME INFORMATION ON:	Viral diseases.
CAN PROVIDE INFORMATION ON:	Diagnostic techniques for serology and viral isolation in avian species.

NAME:	KEYMER, I. F. PhD, FRCVS, FRCPath, CBiol, FIBiol
ADDRESS:	The Old Smithy The Green Edgefield Melton Constable Norfolk NR24 2AL UNITED KINGDOM
INTERESTS:	Avian pathology.
WILLING TO BE CONSULTED ON:	Pathological examination (histopathology; carcasses not accepted).
WOULD WELCOME INFORMATION ON:	Diseases of free-living and captive penguins, including heavy metals.
CAN PROVIDE INFORMATION ON:	Avian diseases.
COMMENT:	No laboratory facilities at above address although some can be arranged.

NAME:	KIRKWOOD, James K. BVSc, PhD, MRCVS
ADDRESS:	Veterinary Science Research Group Institute of Zoology Zoological Society of London Regent's Park London NW1 4RY UNITED KINGDOM
INTERESTS:	Zoo and wild animal management and medicine.
WILLING TO BE CONSULTED ON:	Related subjects, nutrition and growth.
WOULD WELCOME INFORMATION ON:	Abnormalities of skeletal development.

NAME: ADDRESS:	KÖSTERS, Josef DVM Professor Institut fur Geflügelkrankheiten Mittenheimer Str 54 D-8042 Oberschleissheim WEST GERMANY
INTERESTS:	Avian diseases, keeping and breeding of birds, environmental influences on free-living birds.
WILLING TO BE CONSULTED ON:	Related subjects, except toxicology.
WOULD WELCOME INFORMATION ON:	See above.
CAN PROVIDE INFORMATION ON:	See above.
COMMENTS:	Diagnostic materials must be sent only to the Institute address.

NAME: ADDRESS:	LEDGER, John PhD Endangered Wildlife Trust Private Bag XII Parkview 2122 SOUTH AFRICA
INTERESTS:	Avian ectoparasites, especially Phthiraptera and arthropods of potential medical importance.
WILLING TO BE CONSULTED ON:	Parasitology.
CAN PROVIDE INFORMATION ON:	Ectoparasites of Afrotropical birds.

NAME:	LOWENSTINE, Linda
ADDRESS:	University of California
	Davis School of Veterinary Medicine
	Department of Medicine
	Davis, California 95616
	UNITED STATES OF AMERICA
INTERESTS:	Avian medicine and pathology.

NAME:	MACWHIRTER, Patricia BVSc
ADDRESS:	Highbury Veterinary Clinic
	128 Highbury Road
	Burwood, Victoria 3125
	AUSTRALIA
INTERESTS:	Avian medicine—wild and domestic.
WILLING TO BE CONSULTED ON:	Clinical care, gross pathological examination, parasitology, rehabilitation.
WOULD WELCOME INFORMATION ON:	Rehabilitation and diseases of Australian carnivorous birds.
CAN PROVIDE INFORMATION ON:	As above.

NAME:	MADILL, David BVSc, MACVSc
ADDRESS:	570 Springrove Road
	5th Springvale 3172
	Victoria
	AUSTRALIA
INTERESTS:	Cage and aviary bird medicine and surgery.
WILLING TO BE CONSULTED ON:	Related subjects except toxicology.

NAME:	MASON, R. W. BVSc, MVSc
ADDRESS:	Mt. Pleasant Laboratories
	PO Box 46
	South Launceston
	TASMANIA
	AUSTRALIA 7249
INTERESTS:	Routine domestic animal pathology with a special interest in avian pathology.
WILLING TO BE CONSULTED ON:	Related subjects except clinical care.
CAN PROVIDE INFORMATION ON:	Limited histological slide material for comparative pathology etc.

NAME:	McKINNEY, P. MVB, MRCVS
ADDRESS:	International Zoo Veterinary Group
	c/o Al Ain Zoo and Aquarium
	PO Box 1204
	Al Ain
	UNITED ARAB EMIRATES
INTERESTS:	Avian medicine and pathology.
WILLING TO BE CONSULTED ON:	Related subjects.

NAME:	McLEAN, Robert G. PhD
ADDRESS:	Arbovirus Ecology Branch
	Division of Vector-borne Viral Diseases
	Centers for Disease Control
	PO Box 2087
	Fort Collins, Colorado 80522-2087
	UNITED STATES OF AMERICA
INTERESTS:	Avian viral diseases.
WILLING TO BE CONSULTED ON:	Related subjects.
WOULD WELCOME INFORMATION ON:	Related subjects.
CAN PROVIDE INFORMATION ON:	Related subjects.

NAME:	McNAMARA, Tracey S. DVM
ADDRESS:	Animal Health Center
	New York Zoological Society
	Bronx Zoo
	Bronx, NY 10460
	UNITED STATES OF AMERICA
INTERESTS:	Pathology.
WILLING TO BE CONSULTED ON:	Pathological examination.

NAME:	McORIST S. BVSc, MVSc, PhD, MACVS
ADDRESS:	Veterinary Research Institute
	Park Drive
	Parkville, Vic. 3875
	AUSTRALIA
INTERESTS:	Diseases of free-living wild birds.
WILLING TO BE CONSULTED ON:	Related subjects.
WOULD WELCOME INFORMATION ON:	Related subjects, especially wild bird carcasses.
CAN PROVIDE INFORMATION ON:	Related subjects.

NAME:	MOONEY, Nick BSc
ADDRESS:	Department of Lands, Parks and Wildlife GPO Box 44A Hobbart Zoo Tasmania AUSTRALIA
INTERESTS:	Raptor biology.
WILLING TO BE CONSULTED ON:	Clinical care, toxicology, rehabilitation.
WOULD WELCOME INFORMATION ON:	As above.
CAN PROVIDE INFORMATION ON:	As above.

NAME:	MORNER, Torsten Veterinary Surgeon
ADDRESS:	Department of Wildlife Diseases National Veterinary Institute Box 7073, S-750 07 Uppsala SWEDEN
INTERESTS:	Management, care and pathology of captive and wild birds.
WILLING TO BE CONSULTED ON:	Related subjects, except parasitology.

NAME:	NETTLE, Victor F. DVM, MS, PhD
ADDRESS:	Southeastern Cooperative Wildlife Disease Study College of Veterinary Medicine The University of Georgia Athens, GA 30602 UNITED STATES OF AMERICA
INTERESTS:	Wildlife diseases.
WILLING TO BE CONSULTED ON:	Pathological examination, diagnostic laboratory techniques, parasitology, toxicology.
CAN PROVIDE INFORMATION ON:	Reprints, unpublished reports.

NAME:	NEWTON, Ian BSc, DPhil, DSc
ADDRESS:	Monks Wood Experimental Station Abbots Ripton Huntingdon Cambs PE17 2L5 UNITED KINGDOM
INTERESTS:	Effects of pesticides and pollutants on birds.
WILLING TO BE CONSULTED ON:	Analysis for organochlorine pesticides, PCB and heavy metals.

NAME:	ODER, Edwin M. DVM, MAM
ADDRESS:	University of Delaware
	Poultry Diagnostic Laboratory
	RFD #2 Box 47
	Georgetown, DE 19947
	UNITED STATES OF AMERICA
WILLING TO BE CONSULTED ON:	Pathological examination, diagnostic laboratory techniques.

NAME:	OLSEN, Penny BSc and Jerry BSc, BA, MEd
ADDRESS:	RMB 1705
	Read Road
	Sutton
	NSW 2620
	AUSTRALIA
INTERESTS:	Raptor biology.
WILLING TO BE CONSULTED ON:	Rehabilitation, care and handling of captives, captive breeding.

NAME:	OUTLAW, Jennifer BA
ADDRESS:	Louisiana Nature and Science Center
	11000 Lake Forest Blvd
	New Orleans, Louisiana
	UNITED STATES OF AMERICA
INTERESTS:	Raptor rehabilitation, captive propagation of raptors, falconry, carbon monoxide poisoning in Aves, avian Harderian gland.
WILLING TO BE CONSULTED ON:	Clinical care, rehabilitation, captive breeding and maintenance of raptors.
WOULD WELCOME INFORMATION ON:	Raptor rehabilitation, avian carbon monoxide poisoning, avian Harderian gland.
CAN PROVIDE INFORMATION ON:	Will answer all requests.

NAME:	OZVEGY, Josef Veterinary Surgeon
ADDRESS:	J6 Lajos 56/a 24000 Subotica YUGOSLAVIA
INTERESTS:	Diseases of birds of prey and water birds (Anatidae).
WILLING TO BE CONSULTED ON:	Clinical care, pathological examination.
WOULD WELCOME INFORMATION ON:	Surgical methods and narcosis.
CAN PROVIDE INFORMATION ON:	Narcosis of parrots.

NAME:	PASS, David A. BVSc, MSc, PhD
ADDRESS:	School of Veterinary Studies Murdoch University Murdoch, Western Australia 6150 AUSTRALIA
INTERESTS:	Pathology, viral disease, feathering abnormalities.
WILLING TO BE CONSULTED ON:	Related subjects.

NAME:	PEIRCE, M. A. PhD, FIBiol
ADDRESS:	16 Westmorland Close Woosehill Wokingham Berks RG11 9AZ UNITED KINGDOM
INTERESTS:	Avian haematozoa.
WILLING TO BE CONSULTED ON:	Parasitology.

NAME:	PHILIPS, James R. PhD
ADDRESS:	Math/Science Division Babson College Babson Park (Wellesley), MA 02157 UNITED STATES OF AMERICA
INTERESTS:	Avian parasitic mites, louseflies, nest arthropods.
WILLING TO BE CONSULTED ON:	Parasitology.
WOULD WELCOME INFORMATION ON:	Specimens of avian parasitic mites, louseflies, nest arthropods or information on them.
CAN PROVIDE INFORMATION ON:	Identifications of avian parasitic mites, louseflies, nest arthropods, references on the biology of these invertebrates.

Appendix 1: Register of Laboratories etc.

NAME:	REECE, Rodney Leon BVSc, MSc, MACVSc, FACVSc, MRCVS
ADDRESS:	c/o AFRC Institute for Animal Health Houghton Laboratory Houghton Huntington, Cambs PE17 2DA UNITED KINGDOM
INTERESTS:	Disease diagnosis, prevention and control in flocks.
WILLING TO BE CONSULTED ON:	Pathological examination, toxicology, diagnostic laboratory techniques.
WOULD WELCOME INFORMATION ON:	Copies of slides and photographs of typical and unusual cases—clinical and gross pathology.
CAN PROVIDE INFORMATION ON:	Collection of reference articles on diseases of birds, histological material of typical and unusual cases, photographic cases.

NAME: ADDRESS:	REMPLE, John D. BA, DVM Dubai Falcon Hospital POB 13919 Dubai UNITED ARAB EMIRATES
INTERESTS:	Raptor medicine, surgery, pathology, immunology including preventive medicine.
WILLING TO BE CONSULTED ON:	Clinical care, diagnostic laboratory techniques, parasitology and rehabilitation.
WOULD WELCOME INFORMATION ON:	Viral disease, recent work on *Herpes virus* and vaccination. Need livers/carcasses of *Herpes* hepatosplenitis infected raptors.

NAME: ADDRESS:	RHOADES, Keith R. DVM, PhD National Animal Disease Center USDA—ARS PO Box 70 Ames, Iowa 50010 UNITED STATES OF AMERICA
INTERESTS:	Avian infectious diseases, particularly avian pasteurellosis.
WILLING TO BE CONSULTED ON:	Diagnostic laboratory techniques, avian pasteurellosis.
WOULD WELCOME INFORMATION ON:	Selected *P. multocida* and *P. anatipestifer* strains.
CAN PROVIDE INFORMATION ON:	*P. multocida* serotyping.

NAME:	RIDDLE, Kenton E. BSc, DVM Director
ADDRESS:	Abu Dhabi Falcon Research Hospital PO Box 77, Abu Dhabi UNITED ARAB EMIRATES
INTERESTS:	Avian medicine and surgery, raptor rehabilitation, field studies.
WILLING TO BE CONSULTED ON:	Clinical care, diagnostic laboratory techniques, rehabilitation.
WOULD WELCOME INFORMATION ON:	Clinical chemistry—avian norms, avian pox prophylaxis, vaccination in raptors.
CAN PROVIDE INFORMATION ON:	Clinical pathology values, histopathology—raptor cases.
COMMENTS:	ADFRH is a large new hospital for falcons with sophisticated laboratory, radiology, surgery, clinics. Field hospitals in Morocco and Pakistan.

NAME:	SCULLION, Francis MVB, MRCVS
ADDRESS:	Department of Pathology University of Bristol Comparative Pathology Laboratory School of Veterinary Science Langford, Bristol BS18 7DU UNITED KINGDOM
INTERESTS:	Zoo and wild animal medicine, avian medicine and surgery, conservation.
WILLING TO BE CONSULTED ON:	Related subjects and disease investigation in wildlife populations.

NAME:	SOUCY, L. J. President
ADDRESS:	The Raptor Trust 1390 White Bridge Road Millington NJ 07946 UNITED STATES OF AMERICA
INTERESTS:	Raptor biology, primarily rehabilitation and behaviour.
WILLING TO BE CONSULTED ON:	Rehabilitation, housing and caging of raptors.
WOULD WELCOME INFORMATION ON:	As above.
CAN PROVIDE INFORMATION ON:	General raptor biology, housing and rehabilitation.

Appendix 1: Register of Laboratories etc.

NAME:	SOUTH AFRICAN VETERINARY RESEARCH INSTITUTE
ADDRESS:	Onderstepoort 0110 SOUTH AFRICA
INTERESTS:	Avian disease and pathology.

NAME:	SOUTH AFRICAN INSTITUTE FOR MEDICAL RESEARCH
ADDRESS:	Department of Medical Entomology Box 1038 Johannesburg 2000 SOUTH AFRICA
INTERESTS:	Extensive collections of avian ectoparasites: Contact Mrs. J. Segerman.

NAME:	SPALDING, Marilyn G. DVM
ADDRESS:	Department of Infectious Diseases Box J-137 University of Florida UNITED STATES OF AMERICA
INTERESTS:	Avian disease and parasites, especially of Ciconiiformes.
WILLING TO BE CONSULTED ON:	Pathological examination, diagnostic laboratory techniques, parasitology.
WOULD WELCOME INFORMATION ON:	Diseases and parasites of Ciconiiformes.
CAN PROVIDE INFORMATION ON:	The above area.

NAME:	STORM, Johanna Veterinary Surgeon
ADDRESS:	Loro Parque Puerto De La Cruz Tenerife Canary Islands SPAIN
INTERESTS:	Avian medicine and pathology, especially related to parrots.
WILLING TO BE CONSULTED ON:	Clinical care, rehabilitation and paediatrics.
WOULD WELCOME INFORMATION ON:	Paediatrics, diagnostic laboratory techniques, orthopaedic surgery, pathological examinations.
CAN PROVIDE INFORMATION ON:	Paediatrics, clinical care, rehabilitation.

NAME:	TORRES, H. PhD
ADDRESS:	Institute of Parasitology
	Universidad Austral de Chile
	Valdivia
	CHILE
INTERESTS:	Avian parasitology.

NAME:	TUFTS UNIVERSITY SCHOOL OF VETERINARY MEDICINE WILDLIFE CLINIC
	SEDGWICK, Charles J. DVM, Director
	POKRAS, Mark A. DVM, Veterinary Clinician
ADDRESS:	TUSVM—Wildlife Clinic
	200 Westboro Road
	N. Grafton, Massachusetts 01536
	UNITED STATES OF AMERICA
INTERESTS:	Wildlife rehabilitation, wildlife anaesthesia, allometric scaling of biomedical parameters, surgical anatomy of non-domestic animals, educational programme for veterinarians and wildlife professionals.
WILLING TO BE CONSULTED ON:	Pathological examination, parasitology, anaesthesia, surgical anatomy, conservation of rare species.
WOULD WELCOME INFORMATION ON:	Toxicology, surgical anatomy, nutrition (particularly for marine species).
CAN PROVIDE INFORMATION ON:	Related subjects (limited by time and resources).

NAME:	UNITED STATES OF AMERICA ASSOCIATION OF AVIAN VETERINARIANS
ADDRESS:	PO Box 299
	E. Northport
	NY 11731
	UNITED STATES OF AMERICA
INTERESTS:	Avian medicine and pathology.
WILLING TO BE CONSULTED ON:	The Association has a list of participating pathologists who will examine specimens at no charge where there has been a significant mortality and where a definitive diagnosis as to cause of death would help the remaining population.

NAME:	UNITED STATES DEPARTMENT OF THE INTERIOR FISH AND WILDLIFE SERVICE NATIONAL WILDLIFE HEALTH RESEARCH CENTER
ADDRESS:	6006 Schroeder Road Madison, Wisconsin 53711 UNITED STATES OF AMERICA
INTERESTS:	Primary USA diagnostic laboratory for post-mortem examinations of endangered species as well as providing routine diagnostic support to biologists of the Fish and Wildlife Service.
MEMBERS:	THOMAS, Nancy, Endangered Species Pathologist McALLISTER, Harold, Chief Diagnostic Section FRANSON, J., Christian Leader, Resource Health Team (RTH) ROERTEGEN, Karen (RHT) CONVERSE, Kathryn (RHT) ROFFE, Thomas (RHT) WINDINGSTAD, Ron (RHT) SILEO, Louis, Research Pathologist LOCKE, Louis, Pathologist and Head of the Center's Training Program

NAME:	VOGT, Dagmar Dipl Biol
ADDRESS:	Zwickauerstr 5 D-05400 Koblenz WEST GERMANY
INTERESTS:	Peregrine falcon and other birds of prey, behaviour, habitat structure—correlations with disease and pathology.
WILLING TO BE CONSULTED ON:	Related subjects.
WOULD WELCOME INFORMATION ON:	As above.
CAN PROVIDE INFORMATION ON:	As above.

NAME:	WELLS, Susan DVM
ADDRESS:	Audubon Park Zoo
	6500 Magazine Street
	New Orleans
	LA 70718
	UNITED STATES OF AMERICA
INTERESTS:	Zoo medicine, wild bird rehabilitation.
WILLING TO BE CONSULTED ON:	Clinical care, rehabilitation.
CAN PROVIDE INFORMATION ON:	Post-mortem tissues.

NAME:	WILLIAMS, Elizabeth S. BS, DVM, PhD
ADDRESS:	Wyoming State Veterinary Laboratory
	Department of Veterinary Sciences
	University of Wyoming
	1190 Jackson St
	Laramie, Wyoming 82070
	UNITED STATES OF AMERICA
INTERESTS:	Infectious diseases, epizootiology, pathology.
WILLING TO BE CONSULTED ON:	Pathological examination, diagnostic laboratory techniques, parasitology.
CAN PROVIDE INFORMATION ON:	Pathology and diagnostic techniques.

APPENDIX 2

PROTOCOLS FOR SCREENING BIRDS AND GUIDELINE PROCEDURES FOR INVESTIGATING MORTALITY IN ENDANGERED BIRDS

J. E. COOPER

Royal College of Surgeons of England, Lincoln's Inn Fields, London WC2A 3PN, England

PROTOCOLS FOR SCREENING BIRDS
CLINICAL SCREENING

Basic
Observation and examination
1. Presence or absence of:
   a. clinical signs of disease
   b. injuries or external lesions
   c. ectoparasites
2. a. bodyweight
   b. carpal length
   c. condition score
3. Gross appearance of:
   a. faeces
   b. pellets (where appropriate)

Laboratory tests
1. Presence or absence of protozoan and metazoan parasites in faeces.
2. Presence or absence of parasites or cellular abnormalities in blood smears.

Additional investigations, if personnel and facilities permit
1. Bacteriological examination of swabs from:
   a. trachea
   b. cloaca
2. Examination of blood (in anticoagulant) with particular reference to:
   a. PCV (haematocrit)
   b. total protein
3. Examination of serum for antibodies (serology).

POST-MORTEM SCREENING

Basic
1. Gross examination:
   a. bodyweight
   b. carpal length
   c. condition score
   d. appearance of internal organs
   e. presence or absence of fat
   f. presence or absence of food in crop (if present) and/or stomach
   g. presence or absence of ectoparasites on plumage
   h. presence or absence of endoparasites in alimentary or respiratory tract
2. Toxicology-submission or retention (frozen) of carcass or tissues for analysis (e.g. for chlorinated hydrocarbon pesticides, heavy metals).

Additional investigations, if personnel and facilities permit
1. Bacteriology:
   a. heart blood
   b. intestinal contents
   c. any significant lesions
2. Histopathology:
   a. lung
   b. liver
   c. kidney
   d. any significant lesions
3. Other tests—submission or retention (frozen/fixed) of tissues for virology, mycoplasmology, electron-microscopy etc. Whole body radiography (x-ray) of carcass.

The examination of eggs can also be of value. Standard techniques are described in: COOPER, J. E. 1987. Pathology. *In:* Pendleton, B. A. G., Millsap, B. A., Cline, K. W. & Bird, D. M. (eds) *Raptor Management Techniques Manual.* Institute for Wildlife Research, National Wildlife Federation Scientific and Technical Series No. 10, Washington D.C.

Appendix 2: Protocols and Guidelines 187

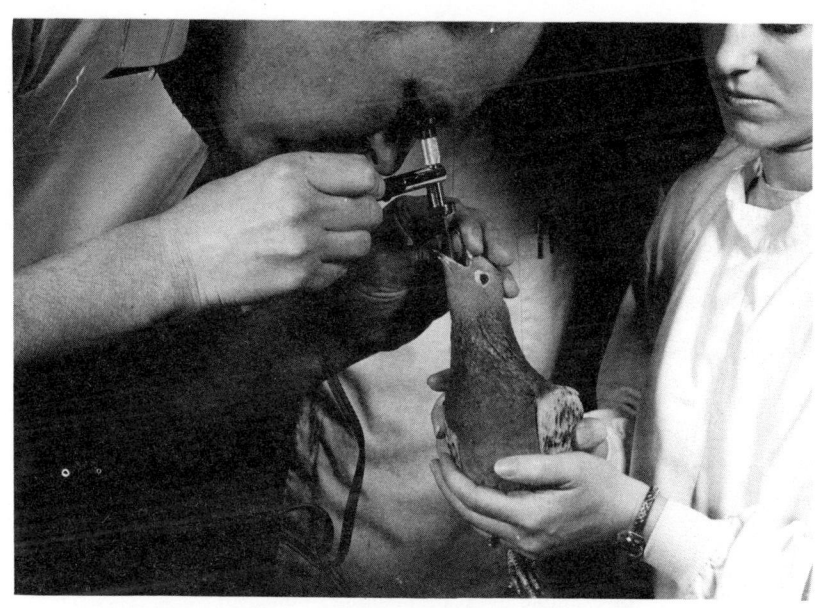

Figure 1: Careful screening of birds is desirable before they are moved from one locality to another. Here, a Domestic Pigeon (*Columba livia*), intended as a foster parent, is examined with an endoscope. (*Photo*: J. E. Cooper)

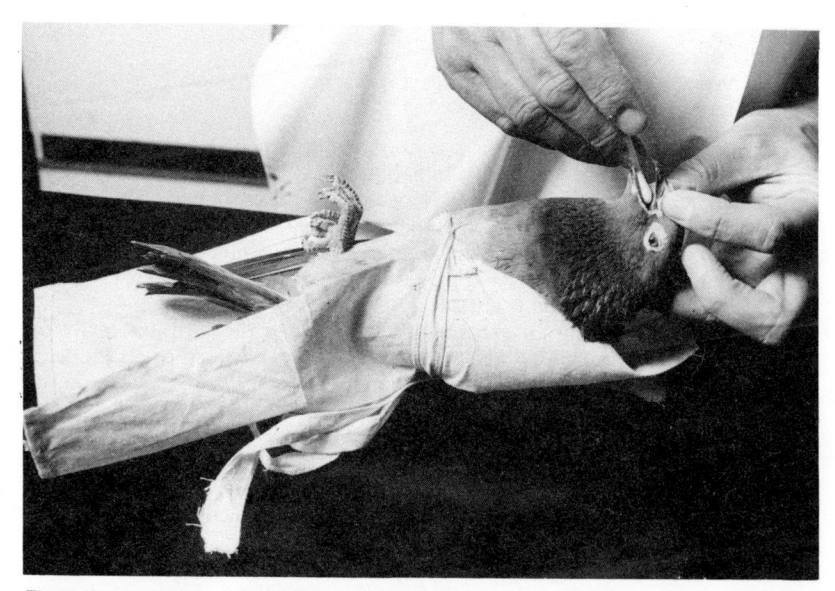

Figure 2: Laboratory investigations form a valuable part of the screening process. A moist swab taken from this bird will be examined under the microscope for the protozoan parasite *Trichomonas gallinae*. (*Photo*: J. E. Cooper)

GUIDELINE PROCEDURES FOR INVESTIGATING MORTALITY IN ENDANGERED BIRDS

If unexpected deaths occur in a population of endangered or rare birds—or even in common species on a large scale—every effort should be made to ascertain the cause. Little is known about causes of mortality in wild birds, and material from rare species should never be wasted. Many factors, ranging from poisoning and parasites to stress and starvation, can be involved and diagnosis may necessitate various tests on different tissues and samples. These guidelines are intended to assist those who may have to deal with dead birds and who have little experience of avian pathology.

General points
If deaths occur:

1. Obtain as much information as possible about the local circumstances of the death(s) and clinical history. *TAKE DETAILED NOTES.*
2. If possible seek advice (for example from a veterinary laboratory or experienced avian pathologist) before embarking upon any examinations yourself.
   If a competent person is available in the near vicinity submit carcasses to him or her for investigation; if it is possible to send specimens to someone elsewhere (for example by 'plane) consider doing so.
3. Pending examination, carcasses or tissues should be chilled (refrigerator temperature) *BUT NOT FROZEN*—although freezing preserves specimens, it damages tissues and can make certain investigations (e.g. histology) very difficult. Freeze only if there is likely to be a delay of 7 days or more before examination is carried out.

Specific points
If you have to carry out a post-mortem examination yourself or advise on procedures:

1. Always follow strict hygienic precautions. In particular, it is wise to wear rubber gloves. Boil or disinfect instruments after use.
2. Keep detailed records. Preferably one person should carry out the examination while another writes. Report systematically everything you see, even if it has to be in non-technical language. Try to have a camera available so that specific features can be photographed, or make sketches—even rough diagrams can be useful.
3. Before commencing an examination, investigate the bird externally for signs of injury, including fractures, and parasites. Check the legs for metal rings (bands) or other identification marks. Describe the plumage, paying particular attention to signs of damage or moulting. Examine the skin of the belly to see if it is red and swollen—possibly indicative of a brood-patch—and if possible try to age the bird: at least ascertain whether it is a fledgling, subadult or adult. Weigh the whole carcass.
4. Dampen the plumage with warm water so as to facilitate post-mortem examination and to reduce airborne infection.
5. Open the body cavity by cutting into the abdomen and lifting the sternum and examine all organs *in situ* before disturbing them (*Figure 1*). Record any abnormalities, e.g. growths or swellings attached to an organ, possible ruptures, haemorrhage etc. Having removed or displaced liver and gut

Appendix 2: Protocols and Guidelines 189

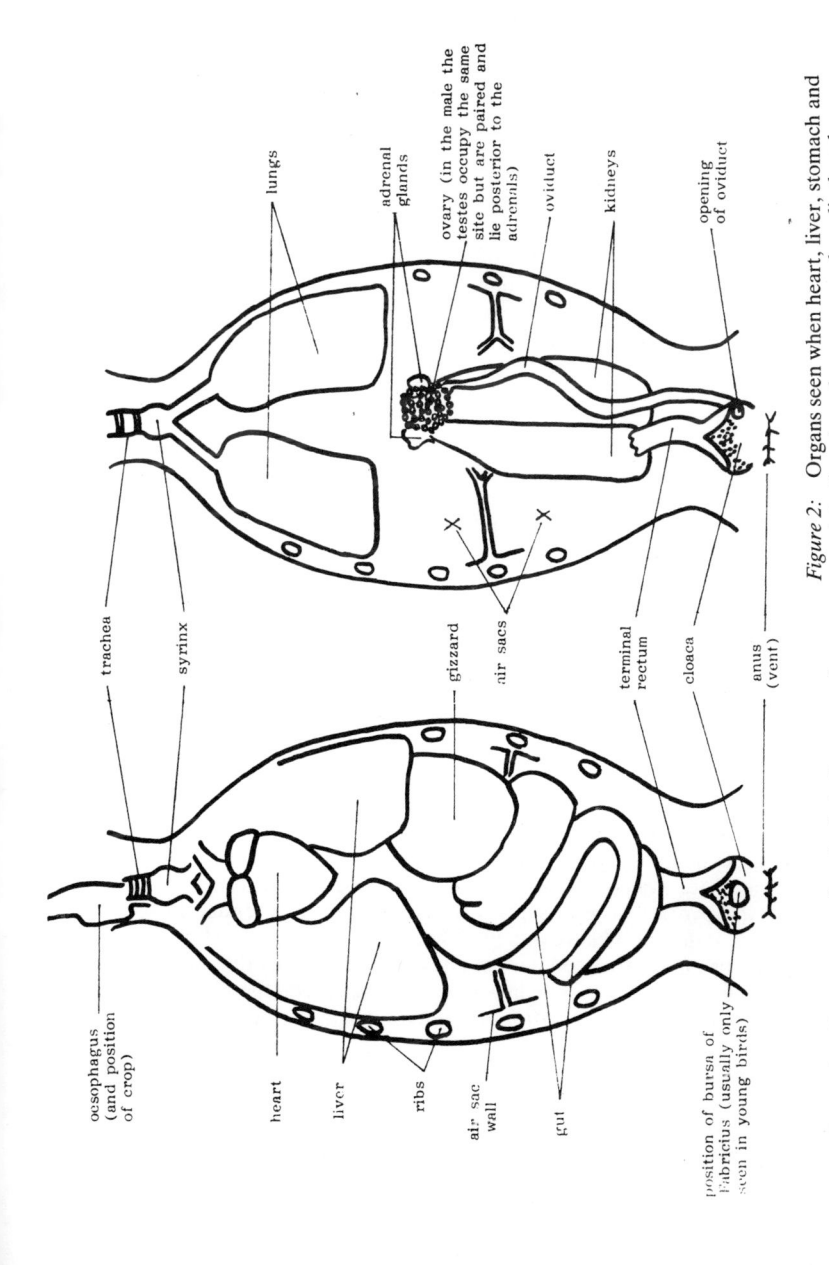

Figure 1: Organs seen when body is first opened.

Figure 2: Organs seen when heart, liver, stomach and intestines have been removed or displaced.

(*Figure 2*) sex the bird from the presence of testes or ovaries and comment on their size and condition (hardly visible, obvious, oviduct containing egg etc). If in doubt, sketch what you see.
6. Take small samples (1cm cubes or less) of any tissues that appear abnormal plus major organs: liver, kidney, intestine, stomach, lung and place them in 10% formalin for subsequent histological examination. If formalin is not available, use 70% alcohol (methylated spirits or high-proof liquor will do in an emergency).
7. Remove the heart and store fresh at refrigerator temperature for later bacteriological examination. If this is not possible, or after culture has been performed, fix the heart in formalin or alcohol.
8. Open parts of the gastro-intestinal tract carefully. See if there is food in the stomach (and/or crop if present): retain the food in alcohol, formalin or deep freeze for subsequent analysis. Search the tract for worms or other parasites; preserve them in formalin or alcohol. If possible, examine a sample of intestinal contents under a microscope for evidence of parasite eggs or protozoa. Refrigerate some gut contents for subsequent parasitological and bacteriological examination; if the latter is not possible add a few drops of formalin or alcohol to preserve eggs and retain the specimen. Similarly examine the trachea or preserve whole in formalin or alcohol.
9. When the points above have been carried out, wrap the whole carcass in at least one plastic bag and ensure it is well labelled (write in pencil or permanent marker and tie to specimen) and freeze it at as low a temperature as possible for subsequent toxicological and virological examination.
10. After examination do not discard anything. Retain feathers, skin, pellets and stomach contents. These can all be frozen for reference at a later date.

If pathological samples have to be sent by post or transported elsewhere ensure that they are properly packed. Postal and customs regulations must be consulted: endangered species legislation (CITES) may be applicable. Fresh (non-fixed) pathological material may only be imported into certain countries (e.g. Britain) under licence.

Comments

The above notes are for guidance only. Variations in the protocol may be necessary, depending upon the circumstances. More detailed guidelines in specific cases are available from J. E. Cooper (see title page for address).

Those who work with rare species should anticipate potential problems and at an early stage establish contact with either a local laboratory/veterinary pathologist or an experienced person elsewhere. Materials that may be needed (e.g. formalin) should be kept in stock. A standard textbook which includes data on avian anatomy and diseases should be available for reference, for example:

ARNALL, L. & KEYMER, I. F. 1975. (eds) *Bird Diseases*. Ballière Tindall, London.
COOPER, J. E. & ELEY, J. T. 1979. (eds) *First Aid and Care of Wild Birds*. David and Charles, Newton Abbot.
PETRAK, M. L. 1982. (ed) *Diseases of Cage and Aviary Birds*. Lea and Febiger, Philadelphia.

Reproduced in modified form from leaflet written by J. E. Cooper and published by ICBP in 1983.

INDEX

A

Accipiter gentilis
    (Table 1) 57
Accipiter nisus 9, 71
Acridotheres tristis 100
Aegypius monachus 53
Aerosol transmission of disease 32
Addling of eggs (see also Eggs) 136
Adenoviruses 47
Adrenal stress (see also Stress) 99, 108
Agar (see also Bacteriology) 41
Aggression (see Intraspecific aggression)
Aircraft, role of in disease transmission 124
Aircraft, movement of specimens by 144, 188
Air sacculitis 17
Algae, spread by birds 125
American kestrel 135–139, 152
Anas platyrhynchos 11
Anas poecilorhynchos 12
Anatomy of birds 190
    (Figure 1) 189
    (Figure 2) 189
Animal pathogenicity tests 12, 42
Animal, Plant and Health Inspection Service (USA) 143
Animals, use in diagnosis 43
Antarctic (see also Falklands) 13, 124
Anthelmintics 34
Antibiotics 34, 42
Antibiotic sensitivity 42
    (Figure 2) 43
Antiserum 42
Apteryx spp.
    (Table 1) 58
Arachnids 125
Arboviruses 125
Arbovirus infections 68
Ardeola ibis
    (Table 2) 58
Argusianus argus 131
Argus pheasant 131
Arteriosclerosis 63, 64, 65, 66
Arthropods 11, 37, 125
Arthropod-borne disease 54
Arthropod vectors (see also Vectors and Biting insects) 117
Ascarid worms 18–19, 20, 63, 65, 66, 96
Ascaridia 20, 34
    (Table 3) 19

Ascaridiasis 34
Asia 71
Aspergillus 17, 18, 48, 98
    (Table 3) 19
Association of Avian Veterinarians (AAV) 182
Ataxia 106
Athene cunicularia 26
Atoxoplasma 70
Australia 36, 63, 144, 149, 151, 156, 160, 161, 165, 166, 167, 169, 170, 171, 174, 175, 176, 177, 178, 179
    (Table 1) 57
Autolysis 10
Avian cholera (see also *Pasteurella*) 10, 13, 25, 52
Avian influenza 11–12, 27, 35
    (Table 3) 19
Avian malaria (see also *Plasmodium*) 27, 69, 77–87, 151
Avian pathogens (see also individual organisms) 1–23, 31–38, 42–48
Avian pox 47, 55, 77–87, 126
Avian specimens 141–149
Aviculture (see Captive breeding)
Avipoxvirus (see also Avian pox) 11
    (Table 3) 19

B

Babesia 70
Bacteria (see also individual organisms) 12–17, 27, 41–42, 44–45, 129, 130, 135–139, 152
Bacteria associated with disease
    (Table 1) 44, 45
Bacteriology (see also Bacteria) 41–42, 64, 135–139, 185, 188, 190
Bacteriophage (see Phage types)
Bald eagle
    (Table 1) 57
Banding (see also Ringing) 26, 79, 126, 188
Bangkok 130
Barbary dove 100, 101, 106
Barn owl
    (Table 1) 57
Barred ground dove 96
Belgium 35
Biologists (see also Ecologists) 26, 53–56, 126
Biodiversity Project 152

Birds of prey (see Raptors)
Biting insects (see also Vectors) 117, 125
Bittern 52
Black grouse 132
Black rat (see Ship rat)
Black vulture
  (Figure 1) 53
Blood 40, 80, 130, 187
Blood parasites (see also individual species) 27, 54, 69, 185
Blood samples 40, 185
Blood smears 80, 130, 185
Blood-testing 33, 34, 185
Blue-footed booby
  (Table 1) 57
Blue peafowl 129
Bobwhite quail 117
Bone, diseases of 7, 108
Botaurus stellaris 52
Botulism (see also *Clostridium*) 12, 42, 44, 52
Branta canadensis 96
Branta sandvicensis
  (Table 1) 57–58
  (Figure 9) 110
Brazil 156, 164
Breeding success 108–111
  (Figure 8) 107
  (Figure 9) 110
Britain (see also Great Britain) 56, 141, 143, 149, 190
  (Table 1) 57
Brood-patch 188
Bubo virginianus 36
Budgerigar 6
Bumblefoot 44
Burhinus oedicnemus
  (Figure 5) 6
Burma 129
Burrowing owl 26
Buteo buteo 71
Buteo spp. 9
Buzzard 9, 71

C
CITES (Washington Convention) 143, 144, 147, 190
Cacatua galerita 63–68
Cagebirds 122
Calcium 101
California 32
Cambodia 129
Canada 116, 125, 156, 159, 160, 161, 163, 164, 166, 170, 172, 173
  (Table 1) 57
Cancer (see Neoplasia)
Candida 48

Canker (see also *Trichomonas*) 18, 98
  (Figure 1) 4
Capercaillie 132
Captive birds 35, 51
Captive breeding (see also Zoos) 17, 86, 89, 115
Captive breeding programmes 9, 26, 36, 75, 93, 115, 122
Carcasses 32, 35, 36, 37, 40, 188
Cardiovascular lesions 63, 64, 65, 66
Carrier, definition of 2
  (Table 3) 19
Carrier birds 9, 11, 13, 16, 41
Casting (see Pellet)
Cataracts 63, 64
Cattle egret
  (Table 1) 57
Cerebellar hypoplasia 95
Certificate (see Licence)
Certification, veterinary 35, 145
Cestode (tapeworm) 10, 20, 35
  (Table 3) 19
  (Figure 6) 14
Chemotherapy 37, 75
Chicken (see also Fowl) 9, 12, 34, 74
Chile 156, 182
Chilling of birds, eggs, specimens 103, 188, 190
  (Figure 2) 91
China 129
Chinese spot-billed ducks 12
Chrysolophus amherstiae 132
Chukar 118
Chlamydia (psittaci) 12–13, 31, 34, 45, 98
  (Table 3) 19
Chlamydiosis 10, 13, 45, 125
Chlorinated hydrocarbon pesticides (see also Pesticides) 186
Chlortetracycline 34
Chough
  (Table 1) 57
Cleft tail feathers 106
Cliff swallow
  (Table 1) 57
Clinical examination 26, 187
Clinical signs, definition of 2
Cloaca 40, 185
Clostridium 12, 44, 125–126
  (Table 3) 19
Clostridium botulinum 12, 44, 52, 125–126
Clostridium tetani 126
Clubbed down 106
Coccidia (see also *Eimeria*) 10, 18, 126, 129, 131
  (Table 1) 131
  (Figure 6) 14
Coccidiosis (see also Coccidia) 34, 35
Coccidiostats 34

Cockatoos 63, 65, 66, 67, 68
Cockroaches 35
Collared dove 108
Collections (see Reference collections)
Colonial birds 125
Columba livia 5, 13, 55, 71, 99
    (Figure 1) 4
    (Table 5) 100
    (Figure 9) 110
Columba mayeri (see *Nesoenas mayeri*)
Columba oenas
    (Table 5) 100
    (Table 9) 109
Columba palumbus 99, 109
    (Table 5) 100
Columbina cruziana
    (Table 5) 100
    (Table 9) 109
Columbina talpacoti
    (Table 5) 100, 109
    (Table 9) 109
Common bronzewing (pigeon)
    (Figure 2) 4
Common mynah 100
Common pigeon (see also Domestic pigeon)
    (Figure 1) 4
Common tern 11, 124
Competitors 37
Congenital defects (see Developmental abnormalities)
Conservation controls 142, 143, 144
Contamination 40
Contracaecum 63, 65, 66
Control of avian pathogens 31, 34, 37
Coracina typica 109
Corvus hawaiiensis 77–87, 108
    (Table 1) 58
Corynebacterium 98
Crane herpesvirus 47
Crested fireback 131
Crooked toe deformity 106
Crop-milk 103
Crop rupture 103
Crop samples 40, 186
Cryptosporidium 18
Culicoides 70
Culling 9, 37
Culture 41
Culture media 41
Curled toe paralysis 108
Customs 144, 145, 191
Cyclones 93, 100
Czechoslovakia 132

D

Deficiencies, nutritional ix, 2, 4, 107
Definition of disease 2

Definition of infection 2
Definition of pathogen 2
Definitions (other) 2–3
Dehydration 111
Department of Primary Industries and Energy 144
Department of the Environment (DOE) 144, 148
Department of the Interior, Fish and Wildlife Service 144, 184
Derivatives 143, 147
Detection of pathogens 25
Developmental abnormalities 8, 89, 92, 108
    (Figure 2) 91
    (Table 1) 95
Diagnosis (see also individual diseases) 3, 4, 6–7
Diagnostic screening specimens 146–148
    (Table 1) 146–148
Disease, definition of ix, 2
Disease controls 141, 142
Disease investigation 4–9
Disease resistance 37, 152
Disinfection (see also Hygiene) 36, 37
Dispersal of pathogens 121
Documentation for import/export 142, 144, 145
Domestic animals (see also individual species) 123, 151
Domestic pigeon (see also Common pigeon) 13, 99, 106, 109
    (Figure 1) 4
    (Table 4) 99
    (Figure 9) 110
    (Figure 1) 187
Dorcas gazelle 111
Dotterel 56
Doves (see also individual species) 55, 71
Duck plague 27, 125
Ducks 37, 71, 123
Duck virus enteritis 25, 27, 125

E

Earthworm 18
East Germany 158, 169
Eastern equine encephalitis (EEE) 26, 47, 115–119
Ecologists 55, 151
Ecosystem 52
Ectoparasites (see also individual species) 18, 130, 185, 186
Egg breakage 100
Egg failure (see Failure of eggs)
Eggs 32, 33, 34, 36, 77, 111, 136, 137, 186
Eimeria (see also Coccidia)
    (Table 3) 19
Electron-microscopy 42, 46, 186
    (Figure 1) 66

Elimination of avian pathogens 31, 33, 34, 37
Emaciation (see also Starvation) 91
Embryo
 (Figure 2) 91
Embryonic deaths 15, 101–102, 109–110
Embryo survival 25
 (Figure 6) 102
Endangered species x, 141
Endoparasites (see also individual species) 18, 190
Endoscopy
 (Figure 1) 187
England (see also Britain) 32, 70
Epidemiologists 37
Eradication of disease 33, 34
Erysipelas 10, 44
Erysipelothrix 44
Escherichia coli 126, 136
Eudromias morinellus 56
Eudyptes crestanus
 (Table 1) 57
Eudyptula minor 20
 (Figure 4) 5
European Community (EC) 143, 147
European sparrowhawk (see also Sparrowhawk) 9, 44
Examples of pathogens 10–20
Exclusion of pathogens 31, 32–35, 36
Exhaustion (see also Inanition) 18
Exotic diseases 77
Exportation 144
Extinction 54–55

F
FRG (see West Germany)
Faecal bacteria (see also Bacteria) 129, 130, 135–139, 152
Faeces, examination of 28, 130, 185, 190
Failure of eggs 100, 101–102, 109–110
 (Figure 1) 53
Falco columbarius 56
 (Table 1) 57
Falco mexicanus 36
Falco peregrinus 56, 93
 (Table 1) 57
Falco punctatus 36, 54, 71, 74, 138
 (Table 1) 57
Falco sparverius 135–139
Falcon herpesvirus 47
Falklands
 (Table 1) 57
Feather, diseases of 3, 47, 63, 65, 68, 157
 (Figure 1) 66
 (Figure 2) 67
Feather lice 99
Feral cat 85, 92

Feral pigeon (see also Common pigeon and Domestic pigeon)
 (Figure 9) 110
Flea 18
Fluke (see Trematode)
Fodia flavicans
 (Table 1) 57
Food chain 28
Food poisoning 125
Foot-and-mouth disease 122
Foster birds 36, 122, 187
Fouling of nest-box 136
 (Figure 2) 137
Fowl (see also Poultry) 12, 15, 34, 37, 51, 71, 74, 124, 132
Fowl cholera (see also *Pasteurella*) 34
Fowl pest 47, 122
Fowl plague 47, 122, 123
Fowl pox (see also Avian pox) 80, 81
Fractures 2, 63, 65, 189
France 156, 162, 165, 166, 168
Free-living birds (see also individual species) 63, 152
Freezing of carcasses 40, 41, 188, 190
Fregilipus varius 54
French moult 3
Frogmouth 63, 64
Frounce (see Canker and Trichomoniasis)
Fulmar 123
Fulmarus glacialis 123
Fungi 6, 7, 17–18, 41, 46, 48
 (Figure 6) 14
Fungi associated with disease 17–18, 46
 (Table 3) 48
Fungal infection *(Figure 3)* 5
 (Figure 4) 5
 (Figure 5) 6

G
GDR (see East Germany)
Galapagos 55
 (Table 1) 57
Gallus domesticus 51, 71
Gallus gallus 71, 102
Gallus spp. 132
Gamebirds (see also individual species) 9
Gapeworm 26
Geopelia placida 13
Geopelia striata 96
Gene pool 36
Geese 71
Genetic defect (see also Developmental abnormality) 95
Genetic manipulation 37
Genetic selection 152
Giant Canadian goose 94, 96
Goshawk
 (Table 1) 57

Gout 107
Gram's stain 41
Grasshoppers 18
Great Britain 36, 142, 190
Great-horned owl 36
Green peafowl 129–134, 151
    (Table 1) 57
Grey parrot 35
Grus americana 25, 115–119, 132
    (Table 1) 57
Grus canadensis 116, 132
Guam 54–55
    (Table 1) 57
Guam rail
    (Table 1) 57
Guidelines 1, 36, 188–190
Gulf 125
Gut transit time 126
Gyps fulvus 169

H

Haematocrit (see PCV)
Haematology 26–27
Haematozoa (see also individual species) 27, 69, 133, 151
Haemophilus 45
Haemoproteus 27, 69, 131, 133
    (Figure 8) 73
Haliaeetus leucocephalus
    (Table 1) 57
Handling of birds 74
Handling of specimens 40
Hatchability (see also Eggs) 86, 111, 137–138
Hawaii 54–55, 71, 74, 77–87, 108, 151
    (Table 1) 57
Hawaiian crow 77–87, 108, 151
    (Table 1) 57
    (Figure 3) 82
Hawaiian goose
    (Table 1) 57
    (Figure 9) 110
Health (see Disease)
Health status of birds 35
Heavy metals 28, 186
Helminths (see also Cestode, Nematode and Trematode) 18–19, 129, 130, 190
Heron 10, 55, 63, 65, 98
Herpesvirus 27, 36, 47
Hepatitis 63, 65, 66
Hepatozoon 70
Herring gull 123
Hippoboscids 69, 98
Hirundo pyrrhonota
    (Table 1) 57
Histological examination 28, 42, 64, 186, 190

Histopathology (see Histological examination)
Histoplasma capsulatum 125
Histoplasmosis 125
Holland (see also Netherlands) 32, 35
Hoogstraal, Harry 121
Horizontal transmission of disease 10
House sparrow 118
Human health (see also Zoonoses) 32, 55, 122
Humanitarian considerations 56
Hygiene (see also Disinfection) 34, 37, 137, 188, 190
Hypovitaminosis A 94

I

IATA 144
ICBP iii, viii, ix, x, 56, 152–153
IUCN x
Identification of bacteria 41–42
    (Figure 1) 42
Immunity 2, 20, 152
    (Table 3) 19
Import duty (see also Customs) 145
Importation of live birds 31, 32, 35, 36, 75, 141–149
Import controls (regulations) 33, 141–149, 155
    (Table 1) 146
Inanition (see also Starvation) 108–111
Inbreeding 89, 105
    (Table 8) 106
Inbreeding coefficient 101, 103
Inbreeding depression 103–105, 111
Incidence, definition of 7
Inclined feet 106
India 35
Indian Ocean (see also Mascarenes)
    (Table 1) 57
Infection of birds 7, 126
Infectious bronchitis 34
Infectious bursal disease 34
Infectious laryngotracheitis 9–10, 34
Infertility 77, 100, 101, 136
Infertility of eggs (see also Eggs) 86
Influenza 47, 122, 123
Insecticide (see also Pesticides) 74, 133
Insects (see also individual species) 11
Intercurrent disease 2
Intermediate host
    (Figure 9) 17
Intermediate (invertebrate) hosts 20
International Air Transport Association (see IATA)
International Council for Bird Preservation (see ICBP)
International Reference Centre for Avian Haematozoa 75, 171

International Union for Conservation of Nature (see IUCN)
Interstitial nephritis 107
Intraspecific aggression 91, 92
Introduced diseases 78
Investigation of disease 7–10
Isolation (see also Quarantine) 36, 37

J
Jackass penguin
    (Table 1) 57
Java 129
Jersey
    (Table 1) 57
Jersey Wildlife Preservation Trust 89–113
    (Figure 1) 90
    (Figure 4) 93
    (Figure 5) 94
Junglefowl (see also Fowl) 71, 132

K
Kampuchea 129
Kenya 71
    (Table 1) 57
Killing (see Culling)
Kittiwake 123
Kiwis
    (Table 1) 57
Koch's postulates 3

L
Laboratories (see also other headings) 39, 40, 152
Laboratory tests 39–46, 186, 188
Lady Amherst pheasant 132
Lagopus scoticus 52, 56
    (Table 1) 57
Land-use, changes in 124
Lankesterella 70
Larus argentatus 123
Law (see Legal)
Leeches 125
Legal considerations 141–149, 152
Legal restrictions 141–149, 155
Leucocytozoon 27, 69, 96, 98, 132
    (Figure 3) 72
Leucopsar rothschildi
    (Table 1) 57
Lice 15, 18
    (Figure 7) 15
Licence for birds, specimens 142–149, 190
    (Table 1) 146–148
Life-cycles of parasites
    (Figure 8) 16
    (Figure 9) 17
Life span of birds 91
Listeria 44

Little penguin 20
    (Figure 4) 5
Long-tailed macaque 109
Lophura diardi 131
Lophura ignita 131
Lyrurus tetrix 132

M
MAFF 142, 148
Maggots 126
Malaria (see also individual parasites) 54, 55, 108
Mallophaga (see also Lice)
    (Figure 7) 15
Manganese 111
Marek's disease 34, 47
Margarops fuscatus
    (Table 1) 57
Mascarenes (see also Mauritius) 54, 56, 152
Manx shearwater
    (Table 1) 57
Mauritian cuckoo shrike 109
Mauritius 55, 71, 74, 89–113
    (Table 1) 57
Mauritius kestrel 54, 71, 138
    (Table 1) 57
Mechanical transmission of disease 125
Medical profession (see Physician)
Medication (see also Vaccination) 34
Meleagris gallopavo 85
    (Table 1) 57
Melopsittacus undulatus 4
Merganser 18
Mergus serrator 18
Merlin 56
    (Table 1) 57
Metazoan parasites (see also individual species) 18–19
Methods of spread 10
Microbes (see also individual organisms) 46
Microbiological culture 27, 28, 187, 189
Microbiological investigation 39–40, 135–139, 185, 186, 190
Migration 27, 70, 121, 126
Migrating birds 33, 35, 36
Ministry of Agriculture, Fisheries and Food (MAFF) 143, 148
Mites 18, 70, 125
    (Figure 7) 15
Molluscs 20
Mongoose 85, 92
Monitoring (see also Screening) 25, 26–28, 36, 55, 68, 74–75, 151, 152, 185–186
Monkey 109
Morbidity frequency 7
Mortality rate 8–9
Mortality amongst nestlings 77, 86
Mosquitoes 11, 35, 55, 70, 80, 115, 117, 119

Index

Mould (see also Fungi) 65
Moult (see also Feathers) 27, 188
Movement 141–149
Movement of birds 152
Mycobacterium sp. 34, 41
    (Table 1) 45
Mycoplasma 10–12, 33, 45, 186
Myxoviruses 47, 122

N

Nasal swabs 40
Natural death rate 8–9
Necropsy 7, 10, 28
Nematode (Roundworm) 18–19, 20, 34, 52, 65
    (Figure 6) 14
    (Figure 8) 16
    (Figure 9) 17
Neoplasia 4, 6, 185
Nephritis 63, 65, 107
Nephrosis 63, 66
Nesoenas mayeri 36, 55, 74, 89–113
    (Table 1) 57
Nest box 37, 135
    (Figure 1) 137
    (Figure 2) 137
Nestling survival 77, 86
Netherlands 156, 165
Newcastle disease (see also Paramyxoviruses) 2, 10, 32, 33, 35, 40, 98, 123, 143
New Zealand
    (Table 1) 57
Nigeria 156, 158
Nocardia 41
Nutritional deficiencies 106–108
    (Table 1) 95
Nycticorax caledonicus 63–68

O

Ocular lesions 64, 66
Observation 7, 187
Oocysts (see also Coccidia) 18, 96, 129
Orbiviruses (Reoviridae) 47
Orders of birds, susceptibility to disease 46
    (Table 1) 44–45
    (Table 2) 47
    (Table 3) 48
Organ culture 43
Organochlorines 25
Ornithologists (see also Biologists) x, 55, 126, 151
Ornithodoros meusebecki 125
Ornithosis (see also *Chlamydia*) 10, 13, 45, 125
Ostrich
    (Figure 3) 5

Owl herpesvirus 47
Oxford Green Peafowl Project 130

P

PCV (haematocrit) 185
Pacheco's disease 47
Packaging of specimens 40–41, 144
Panthothenic acid 94, 106
Papovaviruses 47
Papua New Guinea
    (Table 1) 57
Parakeets 71
Paramyxoviruses (see also Newcastle disease) 35, 37, 56, 98, 125
Parasites (see also individual species) 10, 65, 129–134, 151, 185, 188, 190
life-cycles of
    (Figure 6) 14
    (Figure 7) 15
    (Figure 8) 16
    (Figure 9) 17
Parasitology 7, 27–28
Parasitic diseases 34
Paratyphoid (see also *Salmonella*) 2, 10, 13, 15, 16
Parvoviruses 47
Passer domesticus 11, 118
Pasteurella 10, 13, 25, 45, 52, 98
    (Table 3) 19
Pathogen, definition of 2
Pathogens (see individual organisms)
Pathologists 188, 190
Patuxent Wildlife Research Center 83
Pavo cristatus 129
Pavo muticus 129–134
    (Table 1) 57
Peaceful dove 13
Pearly-eyed thrasher
    (Table 1) 57
Pekin duck 11
Pellet 185, 190
Penguins (see also individual species) 18, 71
Peregrine 56, 93
    (Table 1) 57
Permit (see Licence)
Perosis (see also Deficiencies) 2, 7
Persistence of pathogens 37
Peru
    (Table 1) 57
Pesticides (see also individual groups) 28, 64, 186
Pests (see also individual species) 35, 36
Pet trade 75
Phage types 35
Phaps elegans 4
Pheasant (see also individual species) 12, 145

Philippines
 (Table 1) 57
Philippine eagle
 (Table 1) 57
Physician 126
Picornaviruses 47
Pigeon (see also individual species) 13, 20
Pigs 125
Pink pigeon 74, 89–113, 151
 (Table 1) 57
 (Figure 1) 90
 (Figure 2) 91
Pithecophaga jefferyi
 (Table 1) 57
Plants, spread by birds 125
Plasmodium 27, 69, 132
 (Figure 5) 73
Platycercus elegans 63–68
Podargus strigoides 63–68
Poisons (see also Pesticides) ix, 186, 188
Polychlorinated biphenyls 25
Population dynamics 3–4, 63
Postal regulations 40, 41, 144, 190
Post-mortem examination (see also Necropsy) 9, 28, 188–190
 (Figure 1) 189
 (Figure 2) 189
Poultry (see also Fowl) 1, 4, 11, 12, 31, 32, 33, 34, 35, 123, 142, 147
Poultry products 33
Pox (see also Avian pox and Fowl pox) 10, 54, 108, 151
Poxviruses 10–11
 (Table 2) 47
Prairie falcon 36
Predation 10, 11, 37, 85, 100, 109, 136
Premature birth 111
Premature death 55
Preservation of specimens (see also Freezing) 189, 190
Prevalence, definition of 7
Proteus vulgaris 136
Protocols for screening birds 187–188
Protozoa (see also Haematozoa and individual species) 18, 35, 69–76, 98, 125, 185
 (Figure 6) 14
Psittacine beak and feather dystrophy (disease) (PBFD) 3, 47, 63, 65, 68, 151
 (Table 1) 65
 (Figure 1) 66
 (Figure 2) 67
Psittacine birds (see also individual species) 13, 18, 32, 34, 35
Psittacosis (see also *Chlamydia*) 13, 45
Psittacus erithacus 35
Public health officials 126
Puerto Rico
 (Table 1) 57

Puffinosis 47
Puffinus puffinus
 (Table 1) 57
Pullorum disease (see also *Salmonella*) 33
Pyrrhocorax pyrrhocorax
 (Table 1) 57

Q
Quail (see also individual species) 12
Quarantine (see also Isolation) 32, 33, 34, 35, 36, 37, 143

R
Rabies 122, 142
Racing pigeon (see also Pigeon) 6
Raccoon 13, 20
Rallus owsta
 (Table 1) 58
Raptors (see also individual species) 9, 11, 12, 18
Rats (see Ship rats)
Records 188
Red grouse 52, 56
 (Table 1) 57
Reference centres 152, 155, 185
Reference collections 56, 152
Register of laboratories 155–185
Renal failure (see also Nephritis and Nephrosis) 95
Reovirus 35
Reproductive performance 25, 55, 136
Reptiles 18
Research 58, 63, 152–153
Reserves 36
Resolutions (of Symposium) 152
Réunion starling 54
Riboflavin 95, 108, 110
Rickettsia 132, 133
Ringing (banding) 26, 79, 126, 188
Ring-necked pheasant 118
Rings (bands) 188
Rissa tridactyla 123
Rockhopper penguin
 (Table 1) 57
Rodents 35, 37, 109
Rodrigues fody
 (Table 1) 57
Roundworm (see Nematode)
Rosella (parakeet) 63, 65
Rothschild's mynah
 (Table 1) 57
Royal College of Surgeons of England 90, 91, 112
Ruddy ground dove 108–109

S
Salmonella 10, 13–17, 31, 32, 34, 35, 41, 45, 125, 143
 (Table 3) 19

Index

Salmonella pullorum 32, 34
Salmonella typhimurium 35
Samples 7, 39, 40, 141
Sampling rates 7
    (Table 1) 8
Sandhill crane 117, 132
Sanitation (see also Hygiene) 137
Scavengers 10
Scotland 71
Screening of birds (see also Monitoring) 25, 36, 74, 126, 185–186
Scula nebouxi
    (Table 1) 57
Seabirds (see also individual species) 124
Secondary infection 11, 85
Selection of specimens 40
Semen 35, 36, 101, 141
Senegal 35
Sentinel birds (see also Monitoring) 36, 37
Serology 7, 27, 185
Serotyping 42
Seychelles 56
    (Table 1) 57
Shells, of eggs 16, 32
Shigella 45
Ship rat 109
Siberia 124
Siamese fireback 131
Skeletal defects 96, 108
Slipped wing 96, 107
Slugs 20
Snails 20
Snakes 54
South Africa 124, 156, 170, 171, 173, 174, 181
    (Table 1) 57
South African Institute for Medical Research 182
South African Veterinary Research Institute 182
South America 32
South East Asia 32
Spain 156, 159, 164, 181
Sparrowhawk 71
Sparrow 11
Specimens 39, 40, 155
Spermatozoa 101
Spheniscus demersus
    (Table 1) 58
Splayed legs 96, 107
Spotted dove 96
Spotted turtle dove 13
Spread of pathogens 1–23
Squab mortality 102–103
Staphylococcus sp. 44, 126
Staphylococcus aureus 126
Starling 11, 124
Starvation 25, 63, 65, 66, 85, 188

Statisticians 6, 37
Sterna hirundo 11, 121, 124
Sterilization (see also Hygiene) 36
Sternum, deformity of 108
Stone curlew
    (Figure 5) 6
Streptococcus 44
Streptococcus faecalis 136
Streptopelia chinensis 13, 96
Streptopelia decaocto 109
    (Table 5) 100
Streptopelia reisoria 100
Streptopelia senegalensis
    (Table 5) 100
    (Table 9) 109
Streptopelia turtur
    (Table 5) 100
Stress 10, 15, 27, 70, 74, 108, 122, 188
    (Table 1) 95
    (Table 3) 19
Struthio camelus
    (Figure 3) 5
Sturnus vulgaris 11, 125
Submission of specimens 39–40, 141–149
Survival of fledglings 77, 86
Swabs 7, 27, 40, 185
    (Figure 2) 187
Sweden 157, 176
Symptoms, definition of 2
Syngamus (see Gapeworm)

T
Taiwan 35
Tanzania 35
Tapeworm (see also Cestodes) 10, 20, 35
Testing procedures
    (Table 1) 8
Tetanus (see *Clostridium tetani*)
Tetrai urogallus 132
Thailand 74, 129–134
    (Table 1) 57
Thrushes 123
Ticks (see also individual species) 10, 18, 121, 125
Tissues 36, 37
Tissue culture 43
Togaviruses 47, 117
Toxicity tests 42
Toxicology 188, 190
    (Figure 1) 53
Toxin 12
    (Table 3) 19
Transportation of specimens 39, 40, 144
Transport medium 40
Trauma 65
Treatment (see also Medication and Vaccination) 2, 34, 42, 43
Trematode (fluke) 18

Trichomonas 18, 55
   (Table 3) 19
   (Figure 1) 4
   (Figure 2) 187
Trichomonas gallinae 18, 96, 98
Trichomoniasis 98
Tropical nest fly 18, 96, 98
Trypanosoma 69
   (Figure 1) 72
Tuberculosis (see also *Mycobacterium*) 34
Tumour (see Neoplasia)
Turkey 37, 124
Turtur chalcospilos 71
Tyto alba
   (Table 1) 57

U

United Arab Emirates (UEA) 157, 175, 179, 180
United Kingdom (see also Britain) 32, 33, 157, 160, 162, 163, 164, 168, 170, 172, 173, 174, 176, 177, 178, 179, 180, 181
United States (US) Department of the Interior Fish and Wildlife Service 184
United States of America (USA) 115, 116, 149, 157, 158, 160, 162, 163, 164, 165, 166, 167, 168, 169, 170, 171, 172, 174, 175, 176, 177, 178, 179, 180, 181, 182, 183, 184
U.S. Department of Agriculture 143
U.S. Fish and Wildlife Service 79, 116

V

Vaccines (Vaccination) 9, 34, 37, 115, 117, 119, 152
Vectors of disease (see also individual species) 37, 74, 82, 118
   (Table 3) 19
Venezuela 158, 170
Vertical transmission of disease 10, 16
Veterinarian 3, 26, 33, 53, 56, 126, 188
Veterinary surgeon 33, 53, 56, 112, 126
Viraemia 118
Virology (see also Viruses) 42–43, 186, 190
Viruses 7, 10–12, 27, 40, 41, 42, 43, 46, 47, 56, 77–87, 115–119, 122–126
   (Table 2) 47
   (Figure 1) 66
Vitamin A 94, 106, 110
Vitamin deficiencies 94
Vitamins (see individual vitamins)
Vultures 12

W

Washington Convention (see also CITES) 143
Waterfowl (see also individual species) 18, 25, 52
Welfare (see Humanitarian considerations)
West Africa 35, 124
West Germany 158, 161, 173, 184
   (Table 1) 57
Western duck sickness (see also Botulism) 12
Whooping cranes 25, 115–119, 132, 151
   (Table 1) 57
Wildlife biologists (see Biologists)
Wildlife disease, 1, 8, 46, 151
Wild turkeys 85
   (Table 1) 57
Windborne spread of disease 32
Wood pigeon 99, 108
Worms (see Helminths)

X

X-ray (radiography) 186

Y

Yeast (see also Fungi)
   (Figure 6) 14
Yersinia 45, 98
   (Figure 2) 4
Yolk sac 2, 8, 13, 103
Yugoslavia 158, 178
   (Table 1) 57

Z

Zaire 35
Zambia 70
Zenaida macroura
   (Table 9) 109
Zinc 4, 95
Zoonoses (see also Human health) 13, 18, 55, 68, 118, 123, 142, 152
Zoos (see also Captive breeding programmes) 9, 52, 71

The editor acknowledges with gratitude the assistance of Mr & Mrs B. Milne in the compilation of this index.

ICBP Study Reports

1. Turkish Bustard Survey 1981
2. Bengal Florican Survey 1982
7. Bird Conservation in the Pacific Islands 1986
8. The Fuerteventura Stonechat Project 1985
9. Waterbirds in South-East Sumatra 1984
10. Survey of Houbara Bustards in Fuerteventura 1984/85
11. Bird Conservation Priorities in Nigeria 1985
12. Ornithological Survey of Lake Tota 1982
13. Assessment of Illegal Shooting and Catching of Birds in Malta 1985
14. Results of Census of Milky Stork in West Java 1984
15. Conservation of Oku Mountain Forest, Cameroon 1986
17. Eradication of Feral Goats from Small Islands 1986
18. Bottleneck Areas for Migratory Birds in the Mediterranean Region 1987
19. Cambridge Conservation Study: Taita Hills, Kenya 1985
20. Zahamena Forest (Madagascar) Expedition 1985
21. An Account of the Illegal Catching and Shooting of Birds in Cyprus during 1986
22. A Review of the Problems affecting Palearctic Migratory Birds in Africa 1987
23. Report of the University of East Anglia Martinque Oriole Expedition 1986
24. A Survey of the Avifauna of Sao Tome and Principe 1987
25. A Survey of the Endemic Avifauna of the Comoro Islands 1985
26. The Coastal Wetlands of Liberia: Their Importance for Wintering Waterbirds 1986
27. The Conservation Status of Imperial and Red-necked Parrots on Dominica 1987

£4 each from ICBP

Other ICBP Publications

The Endemic Birds of Madagascar T. J. Dee (1986). 173 pp. £8.00.
Bustard Studies Vol. 1 (1983). 92 pp. £5.00
Bustard Studies Vol. 2 (1985). 188 pp. £8.00
Bustard Studies Vol. 3 (1987). 218 pp. £12.50
Bustards—an introduction to all the world's 22 species of bustards (with colour photos)—a limited number of copies still available. 31 pp. £4.50.
Birds of Lebanon and the Jordan Area. S. Vere Benson (1970). 250 pp. English text. £4.50.
Birds of Lebanon, Syria and Jordan and for use in neighbouring Arab states. S. Vere Benson (1984). 127 pp. Arabic text. £5.00.